BARKLEY DEFICITS IN EXECUTIVE FUNCTIONING SCALE— CHILDREN AND ADOLESCENTS (BDEFS-CA)

Selected Works by Russell A. Barkley

For more information, visit the author's website: *www.russellbarkley.org*

FOR PROFESSIONALS

ADHD in Adults: What the Science Says
Russell A. Barkley, Kevin R. Murphy, and Mariellen Fischer

Executive Functions:
What They Are, How They Work, and Why They Evolved
Russell A. Barkley

FOR GENERAL READERS

Taking Charge of ADHD, Revised Edition:
The Complete, Authoritative Guide for Parents
Russell A. Barkley

Your Defiant Child: Eight Steps to Better Behavior
Russell A. Barkley

Your Defiant Teen:
10 Steps to Resolve Conflict and Rebuild Your Relationship
Russell A. Barkley and Arthur L. Robin with Christine M. Benton

ADULT ASSESSMENT SCALES

Barkley Adult ADHD Rating Scale–IV (BAARS-IV)
Russell A. Barkley

Barkley Deficits in Executive Functioning Scale (BDEFS for Adults)
Russell A. Barkley

Barkley Functional Impairment Scale (BFIS for Adults)
Russell A. Barkley

CHILD ASSESSMENT SCALE

Barkley Functional Impairment Scale—
Children and Adolescents (BFIS-CA)
Russell A. Barkley

Barkley Deficits in Executive Functioning Scale— Children and Adolescents (BDEFS-CA)

Russell A. Barkley

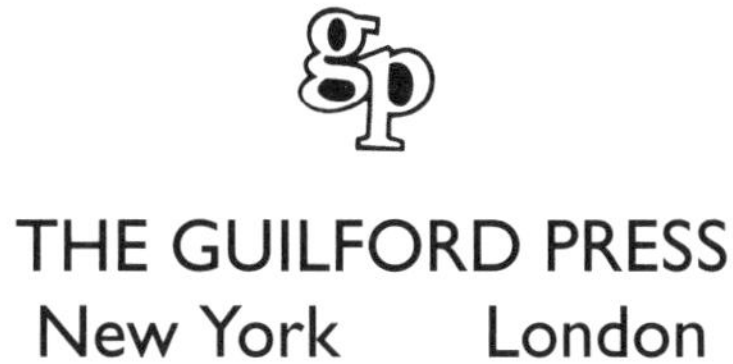

THE GUILFORD PRESS
New York London

For Liam, Laura, and Steve

A Division of Guilford Publications, Inc.
72 Spring Street, New York, NY 10012
www.guilford.com

Printed in the United States of America

This book is printed on acid-free paper.

Last digit is print number: 9 8 7 6 5 4 3 2 1

The author has checked with sources believed to be reliable in his efforts to provide information that is complete and generally in accord with the standards of practice that are accepted at the time of publication. However, in view of the possibility of human error or changes in behavioral, mental health, or medical sciences, neither the author, nor the editor and publisher, nor any other party who has been involved in the preparation or publication of this work warrants that the information contained herein is in every respect accurate or complete, and they are not responsible for any errors or omissions or the results obtained from the use of such information. Readers are encouraged to confirm the information contained in this book with other sources.

Library of Congress Cataloging-in-Publication Data

Barkley, Russell A., 1949–
Barkley deficits in executive functioning scale—children and adolescents (BDEFS-CA) / Russell A. Barkley.
p. cm.
Includes bibliographical references and index.
ISBN 978-1-4625-0394-0 (pbk.)
1. Neuropsychological tests for children. I. Title.
RC386.6.N48B374 2012
618.92′80475—dc23

2011050062

About the Author

Russell A. Barkley, PhD, ABPP, is Clinical Professor of Psychiatry and Pediatrics at the Medical University of South Carolina. Dr. Barkley has published numerous books and more than 260 scientific articles and book chapters on ADHD, executive functioning, and childhood defiance. He is also the editor of the newsletter *The ADHD Report*. Dr. Barkley is well known for his pioneering research on ADHD in both children and adults. His rating scales are based on more than 16 years of research using prototypes of the scales, and are normed on large samples representative of the U.S. population.

Acknowledgments

This manual describes the development, validation, and norming of the Barkley Deficits in Executive Functioning Scale—Children and Adolescents (BDEFS-CA), which can be used in the evaluation of executive functioning deficits in children. The initial validation of the prototype of the BDEFS for adults was made possible with the assistance of Kevin R. Murphy, PhD, Mariellen Fischer, PhD, and others during the more than 16 years it took to develop, scientifically evaluate, and finally publish the latest version of that scale. I am very grateful to them for that assistance and for their friendship over the past 20 years. I also wish to thank Wendy Mansfield and Sergei Rodkin of Knowledge Networks (Menlo Park, California) for their assistance with the collection of the normative sample of parents used to create the norms for the BDEFS-CA in this manual. As with all of my books, I am grateful for the support of my wife of more than 40 years, Patricia Gann Barkley, throughout the research behind this rating scale and the preparation of this manual. I am particularly appreciative of the assistance of Laura Specht Patchkofsky of The Guilford Press for her superlative production editing of the original manuscript. Finally, I continue to express my deep appreciation to Kitty Moore, Seymour Weingarten, and Robert Matloff of The Guilford Press for their acceptance of, support of, and assistance with this normative project and the publication of the BDEFS-CA.

RUSSELL A. BARKLEY, PhD

Contents

Introduction

This manual reports on the history, normative data, psychometric properties, and scoring and interpretation for the Barkley Deficits in Executive Functioning Scale—Children and Adolescents (BDEFS-CA) and its clinical use for children 6–17 years of age. The Appendix to this manual contains the long form of the BDEFS-CA (70 items) for parents as well as the short-form (20-item) version. There is also a brief interview based on the short form for use in unusual circumstances in which a parent is unable to complete a rating scale. Executive Functioning (EF) Profiles are also provided for converting the raw scores from the long form and short form to percentiles for the child's age group (6–11 years or 12–17 years) and sex.

The BDEFS-CA is the culmination of more than 17 years of research and development on identifying the most useful items for the assessment of deficits in EF in daily life activities. Initially development began with forms for use with adults. Now, in this manual, a downward extension of the adult BDEFS has been created and normed for use with parents in evaluating their children ages 6–17 years. The various versions of the BDEFS scales are *theoretically based,* having been initially constructed from models of EF in the neuropsychological literature, particularly mine (Barkley, 1997a, 1997c, 2012b) and those of others (see Chapter 2). But the BDEFS-CA is also *empirically developed* being based on statistical analyses that were used to identify the most reliable and valid underlying dimensions of EF deficits in daily life. Initially, these dimensions were identified in various samples of adults with attention-deficit/hyperactivity disorder (ADHD) along with clinical and community control groups (Barkley & Murphy, 2010, 2011) as well as with children with ADHD (hyperactivity) followed to adulthood (along with a general community control group of children) (Barkley & Fischer, 2011). The BDEFS was then further studied and validated in a large sample of adults, ages 18–81 years of age, that was representative of the United

States (relative to 2000 U.S. Census information). In this manual, the BDEFS is further developed and validated to serve as a parent rating scale for the evaluation of EF deficits in daily functioning in children 6–17 years of age. Not only are the various BDEFS empirically and theoretically based, reliable, and valid, but they are also exceptionally convenient to use. This is due largely to the willingness of the publisher to grant limited permission to the individual purchaser to photocopy the scales and score sheets for use in his/her clinical or research practice. This saves the purchaser a great deal of time, inconvenience, and expense typically associated with the continual reordering of those scales and scoring sheets, as is commonplace in the scale-publishing industry.

As with the adult version of the BDEFS, this manual begins with a brief introduction to the concept of EF in neuropsychology, along with some discussion of the use of this construct in children. I then provide details of the developmental history of the initial BDEFS and its progression to this parent-report form. The remaining chapters provide information on the normative sample, factor analysis, and other information concerning the scale's reliability, validity, and clinical utility, along with instructions for scoring and interpretation of the scale. The information available appears to be sufficient to recommend the use of the scale in a variety of circumstances. These may include clinical practice settings with parents of children for whom concerns exist about possible EF deficits; in research settings in which the evaluation of EF deficits in children is a specific aim, in treatment trials as a measure of response to child- and parent-focused interventions in which a child's EF is of interest, or in school settings in which screening children for possible deficits in EF as reported by their parents is an important objective. I hope you will find the BDEFS-CA rating scales to be useful in the evaluation of EF deficits in children in their daily life activities as reported by their parents.

CHAPTER 1

Executive Functioning in Children

The BDEFS-CA is a rating scale designed to evaluate the major components of executive functioning in daily life activities of children ages 6–17 as reported by their parents. The scale is intended for use by professionals to evaluate any child within this broad age range for whom there is concern about deficits in EF, such as children with neurological, developmental, or psychiatric disorders or those having psychological difficulties with which deficits in EF may be thought to be associated. The scale is both theoretically and empirically based, having been founded on common conceptualizations of EF, particularly my theory of EF (Barkley, 1997a, 1997c, 2012b), and on statistical analyses revealing the basic underlying dimensions of EF deficits of the items used to create the scale. This chapter presents a brief overview of the history of EF, efforts at defining the construct, and difficulties that have arisen in the use of psychometric tests to evaluate EF and its components.

A Brief History of EF

According to theorists (Dimond, 1980), the term "executive functioning" appears to have originated with Karl Pribram (1973) as a description of the overarching functions of the prefrontal cortex (PFC), though some (Wolf & Wasserstein, 2001) attribute the initial use of the term to Butterfield and Belmont (1977). Pribram (1973) stated that "the frontal cortex is critically involved in implementing executive programmes where these are necessary to maintain brain organization in the face of insufficient redundancy in input processing and in the outcomes of behavior" (p. 301). The study of those "programmes," however, goes back more than 100 years before the invention of the term EF, originating in the medical and scientific interest in the functions of the PFC (Bekhterev, 1905–1907; Harlow, 1848, 1868; Luria, 1966). The history of EF, therefore, shows its inherent conflation with the functions of the PFC (and vice versa) such that the attempt to understand EF at the neuropsychological level of analysis is routinely confused with or reduced to the neurological level; EF is simply what the prefrontal lobes do (Denckla, 1996; Stuss & Benson, 1986). Research, however, has shown that EF is not exclusively a function of the PFC given that the PFC has various networks of connections to other cortical and subcortical zones, as well as the basal ganglia, amygdala and limbic system, and cerebellum (Fuster, 1989, 1997; Luria, 1966; Stuss & Benson, 1986). And the PFC may well engage in certain neuropsychological functions that would typically not be considered to fall under the umbrella of EF, such as simple or automatic sensory–motor activities, speech, and olfactory identification.

Among the first and certainly most famous clinical descriptions involving a PFC injury and its associated neuropsychological deficits is that of Phineas Gage, the railroad foreman who suffered a penetrating head wound that destroyed a large portion of his PFC. This injury led to drastic alterations in his behavior, personality, and social conduct (Harlow, 1848, 1868). Like Gage, other patients with PFC damage described in later textbooks of neuropsychology (Bianchi, 1895) demonstrated a lack of initiative or drive, a curtailing of their circle of interests, profound disturbances of goal-directed behavior, and a loss of abstract or categorical behavior. They also suffered emotional changes, such as a proneness to irritation, emotional instability, and indifference toward their surroundings, often superimposed on depression. Impulsive actions, trivial jokes, and even euphoria were noted to be symptoms of lesions that involved the more basal aspects of the PFC.

Subsequently, in his *Fundamentals of Brain Function,* Bekhterev (1907, as cited in Luria, 1966) observed that damaging the frontal lobes resulted in a disintegration of goal-directed behavior, which Bekhterev viewed as the principal function of the PFC. Later, Bianchi (1922) took a similar view of the purpose of the PFC, as would Luria, noting that "one of the essential results of destruction of the frontal lobes in animals is a *disturbance of the preliminary . . . syntheses underlying the regulation of complex forms of motor operations and the evaluation of the effect of their own actions, without which goal-directed, selective behavior is impossible* (1966, p. 224; original emphasis). In time, this frontal lobe syndrome noted by Luria would evolve into an executive disorder (Fuster, 1997) or a "dysexecutive syndrome" (Baddeley, 1986; Wilson, Alderman, Burgess, Emslie, & Evans, 1996). It would also lead to the modern view that EF is largely concerned with goal-directed action (Welsh & Pennington, 1988).

A Brief Survey of Definitions of EF

Modern definitions of EF relied heavily on these earlier views of the functions of the PFC, declaring that EF consists of a collection of neuropsychological processes involved in the maintenance of goal-directed action, including problem solving (Gioia, Isquith, Guy, & Kenworthy, 2000; Pennington, 1997; Welsh & Pennington, 1988). But the functions of the PFC are numerous. Likewise, so are the number of EFs: Up to 33 such functions were identified in one survey of experts in the field (Eslinger, 1996). The most common functions attributed to the PFC appear to be: anticipation; goal selection; preplanning (establishing ends and means); the integration and cross-temporal execution of goal-directed behavior; the inhibition of more automatic actions and reactions to extraneous stimuli (distractibility); the production of delayed reactions; the monitoring and evaluation of one's goal-directed actions relative to the external environment and the goal, especially in novel circumstances; and the overall intentionality or purposive quality of behavior (Denckla, 1996; Fuster, 1997; Lezak, 1995, 2004; Luria, 1966; Stuss & Benson, 1986). To this list some might also add the functions of drive, motivation, will, and self-awareness (Lezak, 1995; Stuss & Benson, 1986). Welsh and Pennington (1988) reduced this list to just two functions (working memory and inhibition) that interact to resolve conflicts or competing action alternatives in goal-directed activity (Pennington, 1997). These and many other authors acknowledge, however, that "EF" is an umbrella term referring to a collection of related but somewhat distinct abilities, such as planning, set maintenance, impulse control, working memory, and attentional control. Even this list is thought to be provisional and quite general.

Why are these functions considered to be executive in nature? Apparently the only requirement for being an EF is that a brain function somehow must be associated with goal-directed action and problem solving and also with the functioning of the PFC. The fact that such functions are essential when faced with novel situations that require new solutions is only partly helpful. Problematic in these various views of EF is that they assert that various neurocognitive processes are essential for goal-directed action yet (1) often do not specify what those processes actually are and (2) do not indicate just what basis or rationale qualifies them to be considered executive processes while others, equally as important for goal-directed action, are not so considered. What makes a neurocognitive process "executive"? It cannot just be that it contributes to goal-directed action, because conscious sensory–motor actions can be considered to make such a contribution, whereas walking or hand movements alone, for instance, do not seem to fit the term "executive" as it is used in the literature.

The definition of EF has also been approached from an information-processing perspective in which the computer metaphor of brain functioning has predominated. Typical of that viewpoint of EF was the work of Borkowski and Burke (1996) and other authors whose work they summarized in this field. Borkowski and Burke described EF as a set of three components that are directed at problem solving: task analysis (essentially defining the problem), strategy selection and revision, and strategy monitoring. Those authors also cited a different information-processing model developed by Butterfield and Albertson (1995) that views EF as one of three components of cognition: cognition, metacognition, and EF. A similar information-processing view of EF explains it as follows: "The umbrella concept of 'executive control' encompasses those cognitive functions involved in the selection, scheduling and coordination of the computational processes responsible for perception, memory and action (Norman & Shallice, 1986; Shallice, 1994)" (Ciairano, Visu-Petra, & Settanni, 2007, p. 335).

A quite different view of EF was proposed by Hayes, Gifford, and Ruckstuhl (1996) using a more behavior-analytic model and particularly the concept of rule-governed behavior (see Hayes, 1989). Their analysis of the terms often believed to make up EF, as well as many of the tests used to assess EF, led them to conclude that

EF is a special subset of rule-governed (verbally regulated) behavior. Rule-governed behavior is behavior that is being initiated and guided by verbalizations, whether self-directed or provided by others. Hayes and colleagues (1996) argued that EF tasks place people in situations in which previously learned sources of behavioral regulation come into conflict with rules laid down by the task and the examiner. Those task-specific rules are competing with behavior that is otherwise automatic and well practiced. Thus the typical automatic flow of behavior must be interrupted and delayed long enough for the person to discover a new rule or select among previously learned rules that may apply in this situation. Yet interrupting a well-practiced behavior itself often requires that a rule be selected and followed that is initiating the delay in responding. And so in EF tasks an individual often has to implement a rule to inhibit his/her usual ongoing responding, even if he/she is only asked a question about the task. He/she must then either select from among a set of relevant previously learned rules or generate a new one. The latter is a verbal means by which we problem-solve by using second-order rules to discover first-order rules. This view of EF appeared to gain little favor among traditional neuropsychologists, who seemed more comfortable using a cognitive neuropsychological or information-processing view of EF than one derived from behavior analysis. Yet features of it would be incorporated into my own model of EF (Barkley, 1997a, 1997c) through Vygotsky's model of the internalization of self-directed speech.

Barkley's Hybrid Theory of EF

In 1997, I sketched the broad outlines of a theory of EF and applied it specifically to ADHD, a relatively chronic developmental disorder of inattention, impulsivity, and hyperactivity known to be associated with various deficits in EF (Frazier, Demareem, & Youngstrom, 2004; Hervey, Epstein, & Curry, 2004; Willcutt, Doyle, Nigg, Faraone, & Pennington, 2005). This "hybrid" theory was an amalgamation of many of the ideas to be found in other theories or definitions of EF but began with its foundation based on the ideas of Bronowski (1977) concerning the unique properties of human language and cognition. These ideas were combined with those of Fuster (1997) on the functions of the PFC, especially his emphasis on the PFC being of central importance for the cross-temporal organization of behavior toward the future. This theory was subsequently further developed (Barkley, 1997c) and eventually published as a book (1997a). Unique to this theory of EF is that it specifies that:

1. EF is self-regulation toward a goal specifically and the future generally.
2. Self-regulation is a set of self-directed actions, often private but not necessarily so, that the individual uses to change his/her subsequent behavior so as to alter the likelihood of some future outcome (to attain some goal).
3. There appear to be at least five of these self-directed (executive) activities being used to choose goals and to select, enact, and sustain actions toward them.

Each executive (self-directed) activity is argued to have arisen in the same manner as the self-direction and internalization of speech described by Vygotsky (1962).

Five such self-regulatory actions were elaborated in this initial theory, each of which is a conscious, voluntary, effortful action:

1. *Self-inhibition.* This represents (1) the capacity to consciously or voluntarily suppress or otherwise disrupt or prevent the execution of a prepotent or dominant response to an event (the response that has been previously associated with reinforcement or has the highest likelihood of being performed under ordinary circumstances); (2) the capacity to consciously or voluntarily interrupt an ongoing sequence of behavior toward a goal if it is proving to be ineffective; and (3) the capacity to protect the self-directed actions that will subsequently occur and the goal-directed actions they are guiding from interference by external and internal goal-irrelevant events.

2. *Self-directed sensory–motor action.* This is an alternative means of defining nonverbal working memory and refers to the use of self-directed visual imagery, along with the private rehearsal of visuomotor actions it permits. Although this consists largely of visual imagery, or the "mind's eye," it also includes the other senses, such as private rehearing, retasting, resmelling, and refeeling (kinesthetic–proprioceptive experience). In totality, this component of EF provides for the conscious, willful reexperiencing of past events—a metaphorical Cartesian theater of the mind. It is the initial basis of ideas or ideational thinking. Yet it also includes the capacity to practice or reperform sensory–motor actions privately to oneself, providing a form of mental behavioral simulation.

3. *Self-directed private speech.* This is the alternative explanation for the verbal working memory system to the one offered by information-processing and traditional cognitive models of EF, such as Baddeley's (1986) phonological loop in his model of working memory (Baddeley & Hitch, 1994). It is largely based on Vygotsky's (1962) theory of the internalization of speech to form the mind's voice. Individuals talk to themselves to permit private rehearsal of utterances, as well as engaging in self-directed instructions, self-questioning, and other means by which language can be used for self-regulation and problem solving.

4. *Self-directed emotion/motivation.* This component of EF is believed to arise from the combination of the first three, in which the individual learns to use inhibition, private imagery (and private sensing more generally), and private speech to initially inhibit strong emotions and then to down-regulate or otherwise moderate them. The individual then consciously employs the other components to replace the initial strong emotion with alternate emotional responses more consistent with social demands and the individual's goals and longer-term welfare. Because emotions are motivational states, this component of EF also provides for the capacity for self-motivation—the drive states needed to initiate and sustain action toward the future.

5. *Self-directed play (reconstitution).* This component of EF is an alternative to the planning, problem solving, and inventive or generativity/fluency components noted in other views of EF. It is hypothesized to be founded on the development and internalization of play and is seen as essentially a two-step activity. The first is analysis, or taking apart features of the environment and one's own prior behavior

toward it. This is followed by synthesis, or the recombination of components of the environment and behavioral structures into novel combinations. These novel combinations can then be tested against a criterion, such as a problem or goal, for their likely effectiveness in overcoming obstacles to goal attainment (i.e., solving the problem). Although this component begins as observable manual play in young children, it progresses, like the other EF components, to being turned on the self and internalized as a form of private mental play. This permits the manipulation of mentally represented information both about the environment and about prior behavioral structures so as to yield new combinations that can serve as options for goal-directed problem solving. It is possible that this component can be subdivided into both nonverbal and verbal modules that provide for fluency and generativity in each of these forms of behavior. Nonverbal, verbal, and action fluencies are believed to arise from this component of EF.

Unlike many prior efforts to define or conceptualize EF, this view provides a specific operational definition of it; EF consists of acts of self-regulation across time toward future goals. The theory specifies five components or types of self-directed actions that humans use for purposive, goal-directed behavior and that become self-directed: (1) inhibition, (2) sensory–motor action, (3) speech, (4) emotion, and (5) play. The theory states that these functions are executive in nature because they are self-directed actions that alter future consequences. Actions that are not self-directed, including any that are used to attain the goal, are not considered executive in nature (e.g., walking, seeing, hearing, balance, spatial orientation, speech to others). The self-directed actions that are guiding those other activities *are* executive in nature.

More recently, I have greatly elaborated on this initial theory of EF (Barkley, 2012b). First, I have now separated out self-directed attention that gives rise to self-awareness and self-monitoring as a sixth EF component. Previously it was housed under the self-directed sensing component. The two components may still be a single function. Yet, given the importance of self-awareness to evaluating both current and future (desired, possible) states that serves to initiate the other EF components, it seemed to deserve separate standing as an EF in its own right. Second, and more important, I borrowed the concept from evolutionary biology of an extended phenotype (Dawkins, 1982) in order to better understand and explicate the profound impact that EF produces in human social living and cultural life. EF is a person's principal means of survival. Its effects can be observed to radiate outward across spatial, temporal, and social distances from the individual and his/her genotype beyond merely his/her immediate appearance and behavior. These extended phenotypic effects-at-a-distance have a considerable impact on a person's adaptive functioning, reproductive success, and survival. In this expanded model, the six EFs described earlier form the Instrumental–Self-Directed level of EF that is most proximal to PFC development and functioning. It represents the usually private, internalized, or cognitive form of EF by young adulthood. But this level is not sufficient to account for how humans employ EF in daily life activities toward accomplishing their goals in major domains of functioning across days, weeks, and months of time. To do that, one must describe the social functions of EF and create a hierarchy of levels of EF that will emerge over the three decades it appears to take the EF/PFC system to mature.

Like models of driving (Ranney, 1994), EF in this more expanded view (Barkley, 2012b) comprises a hierarchy of increasingly organized sets of goal-directed actions that consist of nested sets of shorter-term subgoal/action complexes. These sets and the lesser goals they achieve can be nested together and strung into sequences to accomplish increasingly larger, more abstract, and longer-term goals. Those goals increasingly involve others, through acts of self-defense and self-reliance to reciprocity, on to cooperation, and eventually to mutualism. Individuals also increasingly utilize cultural devices to achieve their goals as they progress up the hierarchy of the EF extended phenotype. These levels, in order, comprise the Methodical–Self-Reliant, Tactical–Reciprocal, Strategic–Cooperative, and Principled–Mutualistic ones that are perched atop the initial Instrumental–Self-Directed one. Seven developmental capacities are argued to arise from the six Instrumental EF components that increase with maturation and permit the movement upward into higher levels of the EF extended phenotype. These are: (1) increasing behavioral complexity, (2) increasing self-restraint (inhibition), (3) contemplation across increasing spatial distances, (4) contemplation over increasing temporal fore-periods (the future), (5) increasing creation and sustainment of self-motivation, (6) increasing use of and reliance on others to achieve goals, and (7) an increasing use of cultural information and devices for goal selection and attainment. Injuries to or maldevelopment of the EF/PFC system can be seen to result in a collapsing downward of this hierarchical arrangement and a contraction in the seven capacities arising from the development of that system.

All of the Instrumental–Self-Directed EF components used for engaging in goal-directed actions are initiated by, directed toward, and intended for the benefit of oneself and one's self-interests. Thus EF is, by definition, *self-regulation for the purposes of one's longer-term or later self-interests.* As noted previously, self-regulation is any action directed at oneself that changes one's subsequent behavior so as to alter the likelihood of a future outcome (a goal) for oneself (Barkley, 1997a, 1997c; Skinner, 1953). The chief executive is therefore *the self*—the conscious sense of ourselves over time (past, present, and future) and also of our needs, wants, and desires (self-interests) as we perceive them to be *over time.*

This expanded EF phenotype respects the fact that the goals toward which EF and its components are being used are largely *social goals and occur in the context of a social group.* Those social goals are being pursued often with others, sometimes against others, and nearly always in the larger context of others. That is the environmental niche in which EF likely evolved, and the problems posed by it are the ones it most likely evolved to solve (Barkley, 2001, 2012b; Dimond, 1980). From this model, I define EF as being *those self-directed actions (self-regulation) used to choose goals and to select, enact, and sustain actions across time toward those goals typically in the context of others and often using social and cultural means* (Barkley, 2012a). EF is a *meta-construct* in the sense that such self-regulation requires multiple self-directed actions (or interacting mental modules or neuropsychological capacities) each of which contributes to EF (the meta-construct). Disturbances or difficulties in the effective functioning of any one type of self-directed activity or mental module disrupts EF. But it does so in a different way from disturbances in other modules. In other words, EF, defined as self-regulation, is not one thing but involves multiple types of self-directed activities.

Executive functions (self-directed activities) are not independent but interactive and probably hierarchically organized in development. The capacity to hold information in mind (working memory), for example, using visual imagery, requires that the individual inhibit responding to momentary external events and resist interference by competing sources of goal-irrelevant information (inhibition and resistance to distraction). The holding of such information in mind can be further enhanced by self-directed speech, or the phonological loop in Baddeley's (1986) model of working memory. Both of these activities (speech and imagery) may then be subjected to mental manipulation (self-directed play, or the fluency, generativity, or reconstitutive EF) to develop multiple possible options for responding to the situation. The emotional restraint and self-motivation that may be required to drive the goal-directed behavior toward the intended goal may be facilitated or even initiated by self-imagery and self-speech. Because a problem can be defined as a situation for which one does not have a readily available response, it poses by definition a novel or nonroutine situation for the individual. Therefore, EF and its self-directed activities will appear to be most needed and most activated when *novelty* has been encountered.

Developmental Considerations

As just summarized, in my view EF consists of those self-directed actions that permit self-regulation. These self-directed actions are founded on preexecutive mental and behavioral activities that are directed at controlling or reacting to the immediate environment and others within it. But during development some types of human action become self-directed to achieve self-change. Those self-directed activities, or EF capacities, first develop as actions that are largely publicly observable. Over maturation, the public aspects of these actions become inhibited or privatized such that the person can engage in this activity without it activating the peripheral musculoskeletal system; the action can be engaged in within the brain just as if it were going to be publicly expressed, but in this case it is not released into the spinal cord for actual execution. A form of private mental simulation of actions results from this developmental internalization of human self-directed actions. That effort at self-management is being done to alter the likelihood of a later consequence (a goal).

The extended phenotype model of EF, like other views of EF (Anderson, 2002), argues that these various self-directed activities do not arise all at once but in a sequence. Most likely, the first EF component to arise in early child development is self-awareness (self-directed attention), followed closely by inhibition and interference control (self-restraint) and nonverbal working memory (sensory–motor actions toward the self). These serve to initiate self-awareness over time—a conscious sense of time, past, and the future (hindsight, foresight). Within a few years, these initial EF components are followed by the development of other self-directed actions, such as verbal working memory (self-speech), emotional/motivational self-control (self-directed emotional states), and eventually planning and problem solving (self-directed play). By adulthood, much self-directed activity is private, being unobservable or very difficult to observe and therefore is cognitive or mental in form (self-awareness, visual imagery, private audition and speech, private emotion regulation, and mental play, for instance). Other self-directed activities may be more public and outwardly observable (i.e., observable self-speech, writing notes to oneself, posting cues or other stimuli in one's work or living space to increase the likelihood of a later behavior, meditating to reduce a strong negative emotional state, doodling various options for solving a problem on paper, etc.), but they are executive nonetheless.

Obviously, the extent to which EF may be deficient or impaired in a child can be gauged only by making reference to same-age peers and to our understanding of the developmental trajectories of the EF components. An EF component cannot be viewed as delayed or deficient in a child of a particular age if that component has not yet arisen, as in infants or toddlers. The assessment of EF deficits in children, whether by test, rating scale, or direct observational recordings, requires that normative information be available for that measure for a wide range of ages throughout childhood development. Such information is critical in permitting a particular child's score to be compared with those of others of the same age in making the determination that a delay or deficit in that EF component is present. Should such developmental trajectories of the EF components differ as a function of sex, then comparisons with same-sex norms for that age group would also be indispensable.

Typically, developmental models of EF have been based on studies employing factor analyses of psychometric test batteries (Anderson, 2002). To the extent that this approach to measuring EF may be seriously limited (see Chapter 2), such models of EF development will also be limited. Studies using factor analysis usually conclude that EF is both unitary (a single large factor often emerges that accounts for a majority of variance, or evidence is found that the factors are at least significantly related to each other) and diverse, involving multiple components (typically represented by smaller, more specific factors that account for far less variance) (Miyake et al., 2000; for reviews, see also Anderson, 2002; Barkley, 1997a; Best, Miller, & Jones, 2009). Less often acknowledged is that some of these factors likely arise due simply to shared method variance, or the use of multiple scores from a single test that give rise to a factor that simply represents that type of test. In many instances, these specific tests of EF are impure, being confounded by other nonexecutive psychological functions such as language, IQ, and visual–spatial and mechanical abilities, among others (Anderson, 2002; Best et al., 2009). On average, four or more factors are commonly observed across these studies, typically labeled as reflecting inhibition, attentional control, working memory, cognitive flexibility, and planning/problem solving. Often the nonexecutive factor of response speed is also evident in many of these studies. Of these, several are believed to be foundational and even inseparable, these being inhibition and working memory (Bell, Wolfe, & Adkins, 2007; Pennington, 1997). In contrast, rating scales of EF behavior in daily life typically identify one or two large initial factors related to (1) behavioral inhibition (cognitive, motor, and verbal) and emotion regulation and (2) metacognition (working memory, planning, self-monitoring, etc.) in children (Gioia et al., 2000; Thorell et al., 2010). In adults, up to five factors may be evident in such ratings (Barkley, 2011a; Barkley & Murphy, 2011), reflecting time management, self-organization and problem solving, self-restraint (inhibition), self-motivation, and self-regulation of emotion.

Because these EF components may develop at different rates, their trajectories over maturation are not identical or necessarily linear (Anderson, 2002). Nor do these components start their development at the same time or reach their apex of maturation simultaneously. Inhibition (and resistance to distraction) is often viewed as being the first EF component to arise. It seems to be more important to problem solving in early (preschool) childhood, when neuropsychological tests are used to evaluate EF development. This attribution of inhibition as the first of the EF components to arise may be the result of the fact that most of these developmental studies do not have specific measures of self-awareness, which, as argued earlier, ought to be considered as the first EF component or at least as developing simultaneously with inhibition. Other EF components besides inhibition are apparently less differentiable from inhibition in the preschool age group (Hughes, Ensor, Wilson, & Graham, 2010). Available evidence suggests a rapid rise in inhibitory ability during these preschool years, with continuing but less rapid improvement during the school-age years. By early adolescence, this capacity to suppress prepotent responses and demonstrate interference control (resistance to distraction) approaches adult levels of performance (Best et al., 2009).

Beginning in the late preschool to early school years, first working memory (WM) and then set shifting begin their developmental ascent and can be distinguished from the inhibitory EF component (Huizinga, Dolan, & van der Molen, 2006). WM appears to be related to set shifting ability despite these two constructs being distinguishable EF components during childhood and adolescence (Huizinga et al., 2006). Both components continue to mature in a linear fashion until mid- to late adolescence (Huizinga et al., 2006) and may be relied on more often in problem solving by school-age children or adolescents (Best et al., 2009) than was evident in the preschool age group. Once the capacity to inhibit responding to distracting events and to inhibit prepotent responses more generally has developed sufficiently, it permits the child to develop and utilize working memory and mental flexibility for more complex problem solving. Later in the school-age years of development, planning, which is thought by some to be the pinnacle EF, may emerge as a more important EF for both problem solving and goal-directed behavior (Anderson, 2002; Best et al., 2009). It may not achieve its apex or mastery until late adolescence. Across all of these EF components, the age of mastery is directly related to the difficulty of the task being used to assess that component of EF (Schleepen & Jonkman, 2010). For instance, even preschool children seem capable of mastering WM tasks in which just a few pieces of information must be held in mind. But when more units of information are added, the age of mastery may shift into later childhood or even late adolescence (Huizinga et al., 2006).

The development of these components of EF as evaluated by psychometric tasks is related to the development of both social and emotional self-regulation—a relationship that appears to increase with age (Best et al., 2009). This supports the previous contention that EF in humans is highly important for social functioning and not just for the performance of purely cold cognitive tasks, such as WM tests or academic performance. However, the low ecological validity of EF tests (see the next section) may limit what are in actuality even stronger relationships between EF and social functioning. Such low validity would argue for the inclusion of behavioral ratings of EF in future studies of EF development (Anderson, 2002). For instance, Vazsonyi and Huang (2010) found that ratings of self-control, a construct highly related if not identical to EF, that were collected at 4 years of age were highly predictive of children's trajectory of deviant (antisocial) behavior over the next 6 years. It may be that rating scales of EF will prove more valid and important in understanding the development of these relationships between EF and sociocultural functioning than have test batteries that are largely devoid of social factors and that ascertain behavior across relatively brief periods of time, often in highly structured and unnatural clinical settings.

Assessing EF: The Problems with EF Tests

A number of tests have been declared to be measures of EF in the neuropsychological literature (see the meta-analyses of Frazier et al., 2004, and Hervey et al., 2004, for a lengthy list of those EF tests used just in studies of ADHD; see Lezak, 2004, for a more comprehensive review). A major premise in many studies and in the clinical evaluation of EF is that these EF tests are the gold standard for measuring EF. As I have described elsewhere (Barkley, 2011a, 2012b), this largely unquestioned assumption can be criticized for many reasons:

- *Most tests used to assess EF were not originally designed to measure EF* (see Lezak, 2004). Many EF tests were originally developed to assess other psychological functions, such as attention, memory (both verbal and visuospatial), sequencing, abstract reasoning, and language. Others were intended to directly assess response inhibition, planning, and problem solving without regard to these constructs being involved in EF. Many do not assess frontal lobe (EF) functions exclusively or differentially (Dodrill, 1997). But when EF is viewed as a collection of various brain functions that include these constructs, or once it could be demonstrated that deficits on the test were apparently associated with injuries to the PFC, these tests were appropriated for use as EF tests without regard to whether or not those tests actually were sampling the *conceptual* domain of EF as a neuropsychological construct.
- *No consensus definition of EF exists that can be used as the standard for determining the construct validity of EF tests.* As shown earlier, EF is a term that is both general and provisional. It is also quite ambiguous. There is a lack of agreement among researchers on the precise meaning of the term (Castellanos, Sonuga-Barke, Milham, & Tannock, 2006; Denckla, 1996; Willcutt et al., 2005). Instead, reviews of the research seem to focus more on listing the constructs thought to be subsumed under the term and the tests believed to evaluate those constructs, such as response inhibition, resistance to distraction, working memory, planning and problem solving, and set shifting, among others (Boonstra, Oosterlaan, Sergeant, & Buitelaar, 2005; Frazier et al., 2004; Hervey et al., 2004; Willcutt et al., 2005). When no operational definition of EF exists, anything goes. This status ensures that ambiguity will abound with regard to what tests may or may not be considered to reflect the conceptual domain of EF.

• *The structured clinical setting is ill suited to assessing self-regulation across time and its use in novel settings.* EF, as noted previously, is most in demand in ambiguous or novel situations, especially social ones, that are often lacking in external guidance or structure as to how to behave effectively in such settings. The individual must engage in acts of self-regulation and problem solving so as to successfully negotiate the situation, solve the problem, or attain the goal (either self-chosen or assigned by others). These factors rarely exist in one-to-one clinical settings in which a child is provided with specific tasks under the guidance and supervision of an adult (Anderson, 2002; Gioia et al., 2000). In contrast, rating scales can be used to capture a far wider range of child behavior across multiple contexts and months of time. Parents clearly possess a substantial body of knowledge about their children's self-regulation and EF that can be captured by rating scales and used to great advantage in the clinical evaluation of EF deficits in their children and in treatment planning for such deficits.

• *Traditional tests of EF cannot evaluate the cross-temporal nature of EF as used in daily life because of their small ascertainment windows for sampling behavior in the clinic (typically 5–30 minutes per test).* EF tests use exceptionally short temporal durations relative to the hours and even days over which children and adolescents sustain their goal-directed activities and weeks to months over which adults are likely to do so. Such a short ascertainment window makes it difficult if not impossible for EF tests alone to capture the lengthy cross-temporal structures of normal human action. By itself, such a problem guarantees that tests will be related only modestly, if at all, to other means of evaluating EF in naturalistic settings, such as by observations over days or by ratings over weeks and months. Ratings of EF in daily life, on the other hand, do sample behavior across considerably longer periods of time (weeks to months). Ratings or observations, therefore, may be better indicators of the cross-temporal organization of behavior and problem solving toward goals in naturalistic settings than might EF tests.

• *Some of the most important features of EF are not captured by EF tests.* Tests of EF do not evaluate many of the capacities believed to be central to the construct of EF (Dimond, 1980; Eslinger, 1996; Lezak, 1995, 2004). They do not capture constructs such as volition and human will, intentionality or the purposive quality of behavior, self-awareness (of self, context, and others), and even aspects of planning (foresight, objectivity, choice and comparative judgment, hierarchical structuring) and plan execution (self-motivation, self-monitoring, prolonged resistance to interference by goal-irrelevant events, etc.) (Lezak, 1995).

• *EF tests do not directly evaluate self-regulation.*

• *EF tests do not capture the principally social functions of EF, such as reciprocity and social exchange, competition, cooperation, and mutualism more generally* (Barkley, 2012b). EF can be usefully viewed as an extended phenotype, as I have recently shown (Barkley, 2012b). This means that EF produces significant effects at considerable spatial and temporal distances and across substantial social networks that influence the survival and reproductive success of people. Among these extended phenotypic effects, the most important for human survival are social activities such as self-interested reciprocity, competition, cooperation, and mutualism (the mutual or reciprocal concern for the longer-term welfare of others). The extended phenotype model of EF views it as a hierarchy comprising these levels of important human social activities that contracts or even collapses as a consequence of PFC damage or maldevelopment. As presently constructed, EF tests do not capture this essential social purpose of the EF extended phenotype.

• *EF tasks are contaminated by multiple nonexecutive cognitive processes.* EF tasks are rarely pure measures of EF and often require various nonexecutive psychological abilities in their performance (Anderson, 2002; Castellanos et al., 2006). For instance, many EF tests are often found to be significantly influenced by overall general cognitive ability or level of intelligence (Mahone, Hagelthorn, et al., 2002; Riccio, Hall, Morgan, Hynd, & Gonzalez, 1994). This makes their results difficult to interpret as reflecting unadulterated measures of EF. Statistically removing IQ from relationships between EF tests and observations and ratings of EF in natural settings may reduce any significant relationships to nonsignificant status (Mahone, Hagelthorn, et al., 2002; Mangeot, Armstrong, Colvin, Yeates, & Taylor, 2002). And it may also account for the fact that some of the strongest relationships noted to date have been between EF tests and academic achievement scores (Biederman, Petty, Fried, Black, et al., 2008; Gropper & Tannock, 2009; Thorell, 2007) or self-ratings of academic performance (Ready, Stierman, & Paulsen, 2001). Given that both academic achievement and self-rated academic performance are significantly related to IQ, not to mention shared method (testing) variance when academic tests are used, this finding is not surprising. In contrast, EF rating scales are typically not associated with IQ (Alderman, Burgess, Knight, & Henman, 2003; Barkley & Murphy, 2011), and so the issue of contamination by general cognitive ability is far less problematic for ratings than for EF tests.

• *Functional deficits in patients experiencing frontal lobe injuries or those with ADHD presumed to have a frontal lobe disorder are often not detected by EF tests.* Ratings of EF in daily life activities or direct observations of EF performance in natural settings are often found to be superior to EF tests in detecting impairment (Alderman et al., 2003; Barkley & Fischer, 2011; Barkley & Murphy, 2011; Burgess, Alderman, Evans, Emslie, & Wilson, 1998; Kertesz, Nadkarni, Davidson, & Thomas, 2000; Mitchell & Miller, 2008; Wood & Liossi, 2006). Given the strong linkage of EF to PFC functioning in the history of EF (discussed earlier), it is unlikely that those patients having disorders of the PFC would not likewise show impairment in EF. This situation has led some to argue, however, that ADHD is probably not a disorder of EF given that the majority of cases show no deficits on EF tests (Boonstra et al., 2005; Jonsdottir, Bouma, Sergeant, & Scherder, 2006; Willcutt et al., 2005), a conclusion much harder to justify logically in patients with demonstrated PFC damage.

• *EF tests have very low or no ecological validity.* In fact, they correlate poorly if at all with ratings of EF in daily life activities in natural settings. This is true in adults (Alderman et al., 2003; Bogod, Mateer, & MacDonald, 2003; Burgess et al., 1998; Chaytor, Schmitter-Edgecombe, & Burr, 2006; Hummer et al., 2011; Ready et al., 2001; Wood & Liossi, 2006) and children with frontal lobe lesions, in people with traumatic brain injuries (TBI), or in those having other neurological or developmental disorders (Anderson, Anderson, Northam, Jacobs, & Mikiewicz, 2002; Mangeot et al., 2002; Vriezen & Pigott, 2002; Zandt, Prior, & Kyrios, 2009). This is also the case both in adults with ADHD and in children with ADHD followed to adulthood (Barkley & Fischer, 2011; Barkley & Murphy, 2010). The results of those studies usually reveal that any single EF test shares 0–10% of its variance with EF ratings. The relationships are frequently not statistically significant. Even the best combination of EF tests shares approximately 12–20% of the variance with EF ratings or observations as reflected in these studies. Yet these two types of measurement are supposed to be measuring the same construct—EF. If IQ is statistically removed from the results, the few significant relationships found in these studies between EF tests and EF ratings may even become nonsignificant (Mangeot et al., 2002). Something is terribly amiss here if different approaches to measuring the same construct are found to be so poorly related to each other.

Additional evidence for the low ecological validity of EF tests comes from studies in which the performance of frontal-lobe-injured patients in tasks in daily life have been directly observed and correlated with EF test batteries. These studies, too, find little or no relationship between impairment in such performances and EF test results (Alderman et al., 2003; Mitchell & Miller, 2008). Here again, EF tests may account for just 9–15% of the variance or even less in ratings of adaptive impairment, primarily in work activities (Ready et al., 2001; Stavro, Ettenhofer, & Nigg, 2007). In contrast, research has noted moderate relationships between EF ratings and measures of daily adaptive functioning in children with various disorders, including TBI (Gilotty, Kenworthy, Sirian, Black, & Wagner, 2002; Mangeot et al., 2002) and in adults with ADHD (Biederman, Petty, Fried, Doyle, et al., 2008), those with frontal lobe disorders (Alderman et al., 2003), and college undergraduates (Ready et al., 2001). And EF ratings substantially outpredict EF tests in the variance shared with measures of impairments in various major life activities such as occupational functioning, educational history, driving, money management, and criminal conduct (Barkley & Fischer, 2011; Barkley & Murphy, 2010, 2011). The totality of findings to date concerning the relationship of EF tests to EF ratings and of each to impairment in daily life indicates that EF tests are largely not sampling the same constructs as are EF ratings or direct evaluations of EF in daily life (Alderman et al., 2003; Shallice & Burgess, 1991). The available evidence also provides a basis for refusing to accept EF tests as the primary or sole source in establishing the nature of EF deficits in various disorders. If assessing how well people do in using EF in their daily life activities is important in clinically evaluating EF, then rating scales assessing EF are superior to EF tests in doing so. Yet the very plethora of studies using tests exclusively to evaluate EF with various patient and general population samples indicates that these serious problems with EF tests have gone largely unknown, unappreciated, or ignored.

This significant failure of EF tests to relate well to EF ratings, daily life activities, or impairment in major domains of life could well indicate that such tests are not assessing EF. This seems doubtful given that many of these tests have been shown to index activities in various regions of the PFC that largely underlie EF. And it is surely unlikely to be the case that EF ratings are not actually evaluating EF. After all, their item content has been drafted directly from definitions of EF and from lists of putative EF constructs in the literature, as well as from observations and clinical descriptions of patients with PFC lesions believed to manifest the "dysexecutive syndrome" (Burgess et al., 1998; Gioia et al., 2000; Kertesz et al., 2000). Moreover, as noted previously, these ratings are substantially related to impairment in various daily life activities and various domains of adaptive functioning, such as work, education, driving, social relationships, self-sufficiency, and so forth, in which EF would surely be operative.

The solution to this paradox of why EF tests and EF ratings are so poorly related lies elsewhere, most likely in the fact that EF is more hierarchically organized than models built entirely on EF tests indicate (Barkley, 2012b). EF tests likely assess the most rudimentary, moment-to-moment, instrumental, and cold cognitive level of EF. But they are very poor at capturing the higher adaptive, tactical, strategic, and principled levels of EF as they are deployed in daily adaptive functioning, human interactions, and socially cooperative and reciprocal activities that play out over much longer spans of time (days, weeks, months, and years)(Barkley, 2012b). It is here, at these higher, more complex, and longer-term levels, that a rating scale of EF can be useful. The reason is that it uses a far longer ascertainment window for capturing summary judgments of behavior over time and is able to capture EF symptoms in their important, largely social, contexts via the reports of the respondent and from others who know that person well.

Also, if the purpose of evaluating EF in patients is to render some judgment as to their likelihood of experiencing impairments in major domains of life activities, then EF ratings are far superior to EF tests. On the other hand, if the purpose of the evaluation is to assess the most proximal neuropsychological EF activities related to moment-to-moment brain activity, as may be important to do in functional brain imaging studies, then EF tests might be preferable. Yet even that point is arguable in view of recent studies linking neuroimaging results to traits that were assessed via rating scales (Buckholtz et al., 2010). Moreover, such tests can be criticized for stripping out important social and cross-temporal elements of EF, which may reduce the validity of the task in sampling any particular EF or its adaptive (evolutionary) purposes. Because of these difficulties, I undertook the development of a rating scale of EF as reflected in daily adaptive behavior. The development of this scale is described in the next chapter.

CHAPTER 2

Development of the BDEFS-CA

The BDEFS-CA was recently developed out of the adult report form of this same scale (BDEFS; Barkley, 2011a). The development of the BDEFS began more than 16 years ago as an effort to develop a cost-effective means of conveniently capturing the numerous neuropsychological, behavioral, emotional, and motivational symptoms often attributed to deficits in EF. A second, related purpose arose from accumulating evidence that EF tests were not the most ecologically valid means of clinically evaluating EF, as discussed in the previous chapter. Having successfully used rating scales in numerous research projects, I set out to develop a scale that captured the major constructs included in the concept of EF (see Chapter 1). For this, rating scales offer a number of advantages over EF tests.

The Advantages of Parent Rating Scales for Assessing Children

The advantages of parent-completed rating scales for children have been discussed in detail elsewhere (see Barkley, 1988; Cairns & Green, 1979), but those advantages can be summarized here as follows:

- *Rating scales have the ability to gather information from parents or other informants with many years of experience with the child or teenager being rated.* Such information is nearly impossible to gather by other means, such as direct observations.
- *The vastly greater experience of parents with their children occurs across a diversity of settings and circumstances that is nearly impossible to duplicate through any other means* (at least in any cost-effective way).

• *Rating scales permit the collection of data on behaviors that occur extremely infrequently,* such that they are likely to be missed when collecting *in vivo* observations of behavior. Such *in vivo* observations would have to be taken over exceptionally long periods of time to capture such low-frequency episodes.

• *Rating scales can gather information in ways that protect those features of an individual's privacy that have no bearing on the evaluation,* apart from the topic of the rating scale itself. In contrast, direct observations or testing of the individual can prove exceptionally intrusive into the daily life of the individual by giving the examiner the opportunity to witness situations and events in the person's life that have no bearing on the topic or objective of the evaluation.

• *Rating scales are exceptionally inexpensive, far less time-consuming, and hence more efficient and cost-effective than either tests or direct behavioral observation methods for many clinical and research purposes.*

• *Normative data may be available for rating scales to establish the statistical deviance or relative position of the individual within the population concerning a behavior or trait of interest; such data may not be available with other methods of assessing that behavior or trait.* In the case of EF, such normative data can be less costly to collect than is the case with many tests of EF whose norms, if available at all, are typically not representative of large samples of the general population.

• *Rating scales can incorporate a large number of items that represent a given dimension, behavior, or trait that can be captured in a far less time-consuming format than would be the case for equivalent items within a psychological test.*

• *Rating scales can be used to filter out situational variation that has little or no bearing on the purpose of the evaluation.* They can do so by asking for cross-situational judgments of the frequency, intensity, timing, or other aspects of the topography of the behavior under study that would be difficult if not impossible to achieve via a test or direct observational method.

• *Rating scales permit quantitative distinctions to be made concerning the qualitative aspects of human behavior* that are often difficult to obtain through other means, such as tests and observations, at least in a cost-effective manner.

• *Rating scales, like tests and observations, can be used for many different purposes.* These include epidemiological research, the subgrouping of various populations along a trait or behavior of interest, further exploration of etiological hypotheses concerning certain behaviors or disorders, determination of the prognosis of clinical groups of patients followed over long time intervals, and serving as measures of behavior change that may be secondary either to interventions or to a change in the status of the individual, such as evaluating the consequences of various forms of brain injury or the impact of psychiatric disorders or psychological adversities.

For these and other reasons, parent ratings of EF deficits in children's daily life activities have an important role to play in research and clinical practice in various psychological specialties.

Disadvantages of Rating Scales

Rating scales, including those of EF, have some disadvantages that deserve notice. These have also been discussed in detail elsewhere (Barkley, 1988, 2011a; Cairns & Green, 1979). The major points are summarized as follows.

- *Rating scales assume that the respondent and the examiner share an understanding with regard to the nature of the item being rated and the meaning of the anchor points or potential answers being provided on the scale for that item.* One such difficulty, therefore, can arise in the specificity or clarity of the item to be rated, as well as in the answers or anchor points being provided for the rating of the item. To what extent do the examiner and the respondent share an understanding of the items and potential responses? The more precisely the item and its answers can be specified, the greater is the likelihood that the respondent and examiner will share an understanding of the nature of the behavior or trait to be rated and the answers to be provided.
- *The generality or ambiguity of the item being rated and the imprecision of the anchor points of the scale itself, no matter how clear and specific the wording may be, can lead to problems in testing hypotheses that require far more precise measurement than the scale is likely to provide.* Such a problem arises as a consequence of the nature of the hypothesis being tested or the purpose of the assessment. To the degree that great precision in measurement is needed to fulfill that purpose or to test that hypothesis, rating scales may be a poor choice of assessment method for the construct of interest. On the other hand, there are many questions or hypotheses in psychology or purposes in clinical evaluations that do not require such a level of precision. Indeed, using excessively precise forms of measurement such as tests or direct observations of behavior is often more expensive and time-consuming than is necessary to address the issue, whereas a rating scale would serve just as well at far less cost and time. The potential problem of precision of measurement with a rating scale appears only when judged relative to the hypothesis being tested or the intended purpose of the clinical evaluation; it is not an inherent and absolute flaw of rating scales outright.
- *Various factors may influence the capacity of the rater to provide an accurate report of the behavior represented in the items on the scale.* Level of intelligence, education, emotional status, range of life experiences, prior experience with similar rating scales, and a myriad of other factors have the potential to bias the reports of the rater in ways that may affect the accuracy or validity of the ratings being provided. For instance, an adult's anxiety may result in an overreporting of ADHD symptoms by that adult about him/herself relative to the level reported by someone who knows the patient well and is using the same scale. The same is true of EF ratings (see Barkley, Knouse, & Murphy, 2011). It is conceivable that this situation represents a true biasing of the rating of the adult such that it is less valid or less accurate than that rating being provided by the collateral adult. Users of rating scales clearly need to be aware of any findings from research concerning the nature of such biasing effects on the type of rating scale under consideration.

Obviously far more research is needed on the issue of the extent to which other characteristics of the rater influence his/her ratings of EF, whether they represent a bias or error in the rating or a true influence on the actual behavior being rated. To the extent that such biases may operate, measurement error will reduce the reliability and especially the validity of the rating. However, evidence already presented in Chapter 1 indicates that despite such potential biases, rating scales may outperform EF tests in predicting adaptive functioning in daily life activities or impairment in major domains of life. Ratings, therefore, may still have considerable value or, in this case, greater ecological validity, even if they offer imperfect samples of the behaviors being rated. The question in selecting a measure is the intended purpose for which the measure is being used. Some purposes will demand the type of data that can be provided by administering an EF test or by directly observing the participant's behavior in selected settings. Other purposes can be easily fulfilled by the type of information to be gleaned from using a far more cost-effective rating scale of EF deficits.

On the Problem of the Subjectivity of Rating Scales

This discussion of subjectivity is taken from the earlier manual for the BDEFS for adults (Barkley, 2011a). There I noted that rating scales are often criticized for using relatively vague references to frequency of behavior, such as "sometimes," "often," or "very often." To some extent such criticisms are quite justified if one is interested in very precise, fine-grained frequency counts of behavior such as might be gleaned from direct behavioral observations or test responses, for instance, on a reaction-time task. Such precise frequency counts may be necessary, in fact, to test certain psychological hypotheses. But at the level of clinical practice and judgment, and for other research purposes for which such precision is often unnecessary and unduly costly and cumbersome, the more general judgments of parents based on their observations of their children have proven to be sufficiently accurate, convenient, inexpensive, and, most important, reliable, valid, and predictive, and to be of great utility. Indeed, research comparing the scores derived from clinical tests, such as continuous-performance tests or even driving simulators, has often found the test scores to be less predictive of their respective constructs as assessed in natural settings (parent and teacher ratings of inhibition and attention, or department of motor vehicle records or reports of others about one's driving, respectively) than are ratings of the individual's test-taking behavior in that same setting completed by the examiner (Barkley, 1991; Barkley, Murphy, DuPaul, & Bush, 2002; Shelton et al., 1998). To reiterate, each approach to measurement has its place depending on the purpose of the evaluation.

But critics of rating scales often charge that the ratings on a scale are more subjective than the responses of the individual to a test. They are not. This is a misunderstanding in the meaning of the term "subjective," I believe. The answers to rating scale items are not "subjective" and thus cannot be besmirched by this assertion alone. Those responses are directly observable, are recorded on the answer form, can be verified or observed by others, and can be studied for their reliability, validity, and utility as well as can any response to an item on a test. The thoughts, states of mind, and even privately held opinions of the rater *are* subjective as long as they remain in the individual's mind and unobservable to others. In that form, they cannot be tested against reality for their conformance to it—that is to say, their objectivity (Popper, 1979). But once a thought is expressed publicly in any form (verbal, motor, or emotional behavior) that can be observed by others and recorded, as in the case of a rating scale, it is objective—it is observable and verifiable by others. The response itself, regardless of the thought it may be linked to, is an item of observable information that can be tested in various ways for its veracity (truth value) and utility. The degree to which the rating actually represents the privately held opinion of the rater may never be known. The degree to which the rating reflects the actual behavior that is to be rated, however, is a different matter and is open to empirical validation. Thus, if a parent reports that his/her child often has considerable problems remembering things that he/she has been told to do, it is not of so much concern that the rating be evaluated for how well it captured the parent's or child's private mental state. More important is the issue of how well the rating corresponds to the level of problems the child actually has in remembering such things. The validity of the rating as an index of the problem can be investigated, whereas the validity of the rating as a reflection of a private mental state cannot. But it is rare that the latter issue is the one under consideration in the research project or clinical evaluation of a patient. It is the former issue that matters most. Even if the opinion of the rater (parent) about the child is false, it can still be observed and studied as a piece of data like any other, and thus it is not subjective.

To summarize, any charge of subjectivity leveled against interviews and rating scales in an effort to disparage them misses the critical difference here between a thought held in the mind of an individual, which is subjective, and an expression of that thought in any publicly observable form, which is no longer subjective. Even if the belief being expressed by the individual is false, it has still been expressed in a publicly observable way and can be verified and evaluated as a datum in its own right. The validity of relatively broad human estimates as recorded in structured interviews or rating scales concerning the relative frequency of specific behaviors is itself a form of information that can be observed, recorded, and tested, as seen in later chapters, for its reliability, validity, and utility, no differently from a response to any test. That is what matters and should be the basis on which a clinician or scientist chooses a method of measurement, not some inherent bias in favor of tests over rating scales no matter what the issue at hand.

As I have stated in the manual for the adult BDEFS (Barkley, 2011a), whether the behavior of a participant is recorded by his/her circling of a response to an item on a rating scale or by a button press on a device or by a verbal response recorded on some testing answer sheet is a distinction without a difference. All are forms of observable and recordable behavior, and the proof of their validity is in the evidence available about them. The widespread knee-jerk penchant of neuropsychologists to assume that a test is somehow more objective, precise, and therefore useful than a rating scale is a hypothesis; it is not a fact in the bag. The claim deserves to be subjected to testing in research and is not a fact by mere consensus of opinion or proclamation by an authority alone. So far, this assumption of the test as a gold standard of measurement has proven questionable for pursuing certain issues or purposes, such as the prediction of functioning in natural settings or the determination of whether a particular disorder involves deficits in EF, such as ADHD. Clinicians, educational/organizational psychologists, and even researchers need make no apology for using rating scales to assess certain domains of behavior and functioning instead of recording directly observed behavior or giving tests so long as the evidence shows that those scales have merit for the intended purpose. The available evidence shows that for certain purposes rating scales are reliable, valid, and useful forms of measurement, in this case of EF.

Developmental History of the BDEFS-CA

The BDEFS-CA is a downward extension of the previously developed BDEFS for adults (Barkley, 2011a). The development of the original BDEFS for adults spanned 16 years, from scale conceptualization and development of a prototype to testing and validating the prototype in research studies that lasted up to 7 years (Barkley, Murphy, & Fischer, 2008) to final scale construction and the collection of norms in 2010. The BDEFS was initially used to evaluate EF in adults with ADHD. Substantial research found that the disorder was associated with EF deficits on EF tests, at least at the group level of analysis (Frazier et al., 2004; Hervey et al., 2004). But at the individual level of analysis, results for EF tests had proven disappointing in that many individuals with deficits in PFC functioning are not found to be impaired on these tests (see Chapter 1). One other EF rating scale for adults existed at the time the prototype for the BDEFS was being developed. That scale was the Dysexecutive Questionnaire (DEX; Burgess et al., 1998; Chaytor et al., 2006; Wood & Liossi, 2006). The DEX was problematic for various reasons. For one, it was composed of just 20 items that were intended to sample a broad range of deficits in EF believed to be representative of a general dysexecutive (frontal lobe) syndrome. This is a rather limited item pool given the number of constructs believed to exist under the umbrella term of EF. For another reason, this limited item pool was also not theoretically based. It was clinically based in its construction, having been founded mainly on clinical descriptions of patients having PFC injuries. Additionally, the scale produced just a single global summary score believed to reflect the "dysexecutive syndrome" and did not yield separate dimensional scores for the set of EF components believed to make up that syndrome.

The initial prototype of the BDEFS (P-BDEFS; see Barkley & Murphy, 2011) was developed to assess a broad range of EF as represented in the previous chapter, and especially my earlier model of EF (Barkley, 1994, 1997a, 1997c). The prototype was then used in two large federally funded research projects on adults with ADHD (Barkley et al., 2008). One of those projects, the UMASS Study, examined clinic-referred adults diagnosed with ADHD in comparison with both Clinical and Community control groups. The second study was a follow-up study of hyperactive children into young adulthood (mean age 27), known as the Milwaukee Study (see Barkley et al., 2008, for details of both studies).

There were 91 items in the initial pool. They were developed largely to sample the components believed to constitute EF based in part on my theory of EF, in part on a review of the literature regarding the conceptualization of EF and its components, and to some degree on my own more than 20 years of clinical and research experience as a board-certified clinical neuropsychologist at the time of item development. Items were especially drawn from my earlier model of EF and its components (Barkley, 1997a). These included inhibition; nonverbal working memory (self-directed sensing, especially visual imagery); the cross-temporal organization of behavior (sense of time, time management, planning and anticipation); verbal working memory (self-directed private speech, verbal contemplation of one's behavior before acting, etc.); motivational self-regulation (motivating oneself during boring activities, etc.); and reconstitution or fluency (generativity, problem solving, and goal-directed inventiveness), which reflects the ability to develop multiple possible responses to problems. Some additional items were also generated from a review of more than 200 charts of adults diagnosed with ADHD at a regional medical center adult ADHD clinic. That was done because ADHD is largely a disorder of PFC functioning (Bush, Valera, & Seidman, 2005; Hutchinson, Mathias, & Banich, 2008; Mackie et al., 2007; Paloyelis, Mehta, Kuntsi, & Asherson, 2007; Valera, Faraone, Murray, & Seidman, 2007), has long been construed as such (Pontius, 1973), and is characterized by many theorists as being a disorder involving EF (Barkley, 1997c; Castellanos et al., 2006; Nigg & Casey, 2005; Sagvolden, Johansen, Aase, & Russell, 2005). Symptoms of ADHD, as shown in DSM-IV, were intentionally excluded from the scale to avoid contaminating the scale with such items and to permit the study of EF separate from the conceptualization of ADHD.

The scale items focused on problematic symptoms (deficit measurement) rather than on positive or normative EF. The BDEFS was not intended to assess the broad variation of EF in the general population in order to identify the range of individual differences in normal functioning that may exist in that population. Scales focusing on typical EF in a general population may be quite useful in studying the range of individual differences, as in studies of behavior genetics, normal development across the lifespan, or other purposes in which normal variation in a psychological trait is of interest. But the BDEFS was intended for clinical purposes, to be used to evaluate the range of EF deficits in clinic-referred or high-risk adults; that is, to assess symptoms of executive dysfunctioning. The clinician is faced with the question of the extent to which the complaints of a clinical patient concerning problems in EF are indicative of significant difficulties in EF. The question here is how atypical the complaints of the patient are rather than where the person is situated within the distribution of typical variation in EF in the general population.

Deficit or symptom measurement is typical in the development of clinical assessment devices for children having psychological problems, such as the Child Behavior Checklist (Achenbach, 2001), Behavior Assessment System for Children—Second Edition (BASC-2; Reynolds & Kamphaus, 2004), or other rating scales of child EF, such as the Behavior Rating Inventory of Executive Functioning (BRIEF; Gioia et al., 2000; Roth, Isquith, & Gioia, 2005) and the Childhood Executive Functioning Inventory (CHEXI; Thorell & Nyberg, 2008). The distribution of such scores on symptom checklists will be quite different than would the more typical bell-shaped curve of the distribution of normal variation in a typical psychological ability, such as intelligence or academic achievement. The score distribution of the former deficit (symptom) measurement tool can be expected to be highly skewed toward the zero point or low score on the scale, with a steep drop in the percentage of the general population that manifests an increasing number of symptoms. Deficit or symptom assessment evaluates the likelihood that the complaints of a patient are sufficiently severe or numerous as to place the patient significantly outside the distribution of typical complaints for the general population. This is the purpose of the BDEFS and its construction, using items reflecting symptoms or deficits rather than reflecting the range of normal abilities.

Three separate instruments were developed from the original 91-item pool: two were adult rating scales (self- and other-reports), and one was an interview to be given by a clinician. These items were cast in the form of a rating scale to be completed by the participants. This same scale was also recast in a third-person form that would be completed by someone who knew the participant well. This was typically a parent or cohabiting partner, but if that person were not available, a sibling or a close friend was used instead. Each item on these two scales was answered on a 0–3 Likert scale (0, *rarely or not at all,* 1, *sometimes,* 2, *often,* and 3, *very often*). The interview contained the same items as did the rating scale. The measures differed, however, in that the interview items asked only whether the individual had experienced that symptom as occurring "often or more frequently" rather than providing a choice of four possible ratings, as was the case with the rating scale. The term "often" was chosen to signify a symptom because of our earlier work with an adult ADHD rating scale that suggested that this response occurs infrequently in the general population of adults and so can serve as a marker for a problem or symptom (Barkley & Murphy, 2006; Murphy & Barkley, 1996). These instruments served as prototypes for the adult BDEFS.

Identifying Underlying Dimensions of EF in Daily Life Activities

A principal-components factor analysis was applied to the 91 original EF items on the prototype (P-BDEFS; Barkley & Murphy, 2011). Five factors had at least 10 items with their highest loading on a factor; these accounted for at least 2% or more of the variance before rotation (and, incidentally, had eigenvalues of 1.8 or higher). There were 88 items that had loadings of at least .400 on any of these five factors. Three items were dropped from the scale because they did not have a loading of ≥ .400 on any of the final five factors in that analysis (inability to sustain friendships, having poor or sloppy handwriting, and being less able than others to recall events from childhood).

The final five factors (after the varimax rotation) were:

- *Factor 1* (*Self-Management to Time*): the highest-loading items dealt with sense of time, time management, planning, preparing for deadlines, and other goal-directed behavior.

- *Factor 2* (*Self-Organization/Problem Solving*): items pertained to organizing one's thoughts, actions, and writing, thinking quickly when encountering unexpected events, and inventing solutions to problems or obstacles encountered while pursuing goals.

- *Factor 3* (*Self-Discipline* or *Inhibition*): items concerned making impulsive comments, poor inhibition of reactions to events, impulsive decision making, doing things without regard to their consequences, and not thinking about the relevant past or future before acting. A few items also dealt with poor self-awareness and the inability to take other people's perspectives about one's own behavior or a situation.

- *Factor 4* (*Self-Motivation*): items mainly dealing with taking shortcuts in one's work, not doing all assigned work, being described as lazy by others, not putting in much effort on work, needing more supervision than others while working, getting bored easily, and so forth.

- Factor 5 (*Self-Activation/Concentration*): items concerning being easily distracted by one's thoughts when doing boring work; staying awake and alert while working; being able to persist in boring activities; sustained concentration to reading, paperwork, meetings, or other activities that were not interesting; being prone to daydreaming when one should be concentrating; and having to reread uninteresting written material in order to comprehend it.

A factor analysis was also conducted on the version of this rating scale completed by others (Barkley & Murphy, 2011). The same five-factor solution emerged with nearly identical item content. This same factor structure was also found in the analysis of the P-BDEFS interview (Barkley & Fischer, 2011).

Five subscales were created from the P-BDEFS reflecting these factors and composed of just those items having their highest loadings on that scale. For each problem scale, a total score was created based on the sum of the individual raw item scores for that scale. The scales were significantly intercorrelated, ranging from .74 to .88 for the self-ratings and .75 to .88 for the other-ratings. This means that the scales shared 56–77% of their variance, which may indicate the possible existence of a single underlying metaconstruct of deficits in EF (Barkley & Murphy, 2011).

The self-ratings were only modestly related to age (r's ranging from –.11 to –.27), with older individuals having fewer deficits in EF in daily life (Barkley, 2011a). Only one of the scales was modestly but significantly correlated with participant IQ: the Self-Organization/Problem Solving scale ($r = -.15$, $p = .007$) (Barkley & Murphy, 2011). Therefore, this scale shares just 2.9% of its variance with the IQ measure. Results (see Barkley & Murphy, 2011) indicated that the adults with ADHD rated themselves as having significantly more severe EF deficits on all five scales compared with the Clinical and the Community control groups. The Clinical group also rated themselves as having more severe EF deficits than did the Community group. This was also the case for the other-ratings. In the ADHD group, 89–98% fell into the clinically impaired range, as did 83–93% of the Clinical group (7th percentile of the Community group), compared with just 7–11% of the Community group on the five subscales. The ADHD group had a higher percentage rated as impaired on the other ratings on four of the five scales, the exception being the Self-Organization/Problem Solving scale.

The prototype of the BDEFS thus appeared to have utility for the clinical assessment of EF in daily life activities. The initial scale assessed five dimensions of EF deficits in daily life activities and was found to be useful in identifying such deficits in ADHD and other clinically referred adults relative to a Community group, as well as in children with ADHD followed to adulthood. These promising initial results led to further development of the scale, the collection of norms for the final version of the BDEFS, and publication of that information (Barkley, 2011a).

For the final version of the BDEFS, the items from the prototype that were found to have factor loadings of at least .500 or greater on one of the five factors in our earlier study (Barkley & Murphy, 2010) were retained. Therefore, a few items on each of the P-BDEFS scales were abandoned in an attempt to reduce the scale length and hence the time needed to complete the scale without loss of information. One domain of EF appeared to be substantially underrepresented in the original scale and so did not have an opportunity to emerge in the foregoing analyses: the self-regulation of emotion. This is an important component of EF that is often neglected in developing EF test batteries but that appears to be a commonplace observation of the deficits in clinical patients associated with PFC injuries (see Chapter 1).

Research suggests that emotional self-control can be usefully conceptualized as involving a two-stage process: (1) the inhibition of strong emotional reactions to events and (2) the subsequent engagement of self-regulatory actions and strategies. Those strategies include self-soothing, refocusing attention away from the provocative event, reducing and moderating the initial emotion, and organizing the eventual emotional expression so that it is more consistent with and supportive of individual goals and long-term welfare (Barkley, 2010; Gottman & Katz, 1989; Martel, 2009; Masters, 1991; Melnick & Hinshaw, 2000). The modal model of emotional self-regulation developed by Gross (1998; Gross & John, 2003; Gross & Thompson, 2007) was used to generate an additional 10 items to reflect these problems with poor self-regulation of emotional states. Two additional items related to self-motivation were added to evaluate that aspect of EF more completely. This was done in an effort to strengthen (lengthen) the item content of the self-motivation subscale in the P-BDEFS. Gross (1998) argued that there are five sets of emotion regulation strategies: (1) situation selection, (2) situation modification, (3) attention deployment (such as distraction or gaze aversion), (4) cognitive change (such as conscious reappraisal), and (5) response modulation (such as suppressing expressions). These five sets of strategies can be further subdivided according to whether they are antecedent-focused or response-focused. Efforts were made to include at least one item to evaluate each of these five strategies.

This modification of the P-BDEFS was successful in that a subsequent factor analysis of the normative sample of more than 1,200 adults revealed a five-factor solution, one of which was a dimension reflecting the Self-Regulation of Emotion items (Barkley, 2011a). The other four factors were the same as the first four found in the prototype: Self-Management to Time, Self-Organization/Problem Solving, Self-Restraint (inhibition), and Self-Motivation. Only the Self-Activation/Concentration factor failed to replicate in the adult normative sample (Barkley, 2011a). Following further analyses using that normative sample, the final scale was reduced to 89 items (Barkley, 2011a) comprising these five factors: Self-Management to Time, Self-Organization/Problem Solving, Self-Restraint, Self-Motivation, and Self-Regulation of Emotion. The Self-Discipline scale on the original prototype was renamed Self-Restraint to more accurately reflect its focus on the domain of inhibition absent any connotations about self-punishment the former term may have contained.

Those 89 items that were published in the final adult version of the BDEFS (Barkley, 2011a) served as the basis for creating the current parent form of the BDEFS-CA described in this manual. To create that scale, the 14 items that had the highest loading on each subscale were chosen to represent that same subscale on the BDEFS-CA. This created a 70-item scale for parents. It also reduced the time needed to complete the scale, with little if any loss of information contained on each dimension or subscale. Hence the parent form of the BDEFS described in this manual (the BDEFS-CA) was initially based on these 70 items. The wording of each item was then changed from the first to the third person so parents could report about their children. Also, the phrasing of each item was examined for its appropriateness for children and adolescents. Where necessary, items were rephrased to suit these developmental stages. For instance, any time an item referred to work, it was rephrased to refer to schoolwork or work done at home. The ascertainment window given to parents for completing these items was the same as that used in the adult BDEFS—individuals were asked to rate the occurrence of each item based on the previous 6 months. The four anchor points for rating each item were also retained, these being *not at all or rarely, sometimes, often,* and *very often.* Parents were also instructed that if their child was taking any medication for a psychiatric or psychological disorder, they were to rate the child's behavior based on how the child behaved off of his/her medication.

The next chapter describes the characteristics of the U.S. representative sample of parents who complete the BDEFS-CA on children ages 6–17 years.

CHAPTER 3

Normative Sample

The BDEFS-CA was normed on a large, nationally representative sample of 1,922 parents in the United States who had children between the ages of 6 and 17. Consideration was given to geographic regions (nine), socioeconomic status (education, income, and work categories), and ethnic grouping. A national survey company, Knowledge Networks of Menlo Park, California, was hired to conduct the collection of the rating scale data on the sample (see *www.knowledgenetworks.com* for more information on the company).

Methods

Knowledge Networks conducted the survey using the Web-enabled Knowledge Panel®, a probability-based panel designed to be representative of the U.S. population. Initially, participants were chosen scientifically through random selection of telephone numbers and residential addresses. Persons in selected households were then invited by telephone or by mail to participate in the Knowledge Panel. For those who agreed to participate but did not already have Internet access, Knowledge Networks provided a laptop and Internet service provider connection at no cost. People who already had computers and Internet service were permitted to participate using their own equipment. Panelists then received unique log-in information about accessing surveys online and were sent emails throughout each month inviting them to participate in research. Panelists were paid for their completion of the survey. More technical information is available at *www.knowledgenetworks.com/ganp/reviewer-info.html.*

The BDEFS-CA was uploaded to an Internet site to which members of the Knowledge Panel had access. Of the total of 1,922 parents who completed the scale,

48.4% had one child in this age range. The remainder had two or more children in that age range. The mean number of children per family in the age range for qualification was 1.7 (*SD* = 0.87), with a range from 1 to 9. Parents who had more than one child in this age range entered the ages and sex of each of the children who were in this range. One child was then randomly chosen by a Knowledge Networks algorithm to be the target of the rating scale. The survey was conducted in August of 2011 and was completed within 3 weeks of the initial invitation.

The BDEFS-CA was given to Knowledge Networks as a rating scale on which parents were to answer each item using a 4-point (1–4) Likert scale of 1 = *rarely or not at all*, 2 = *sometimes*, 3 = *often*, and 4 = *very often*. Knowledge Networks requires that participants (parents) be given the option of choosing not to answer a question. Most participants did answer every one. Rarely, for some questions, a participant did refuse to answer the question. For each of the questions for which refusals occurred, the refusal rate ranged from 0.2 to 1.7%, averaging approximately 1.0% as the refusal rate per item. In these rare cases, the missing answer was replaced with a 1, the lowest rating, so that all of the remaining data for these participants could be used in the project. This practice was based on the rationale that this would create a conservative bias in these few unanswered responses to each item.

Demographic Characteristics of the National Sample

Knowledge Networks was originally contracted to obtain completed scales on at least 1,800 children, broken down into 12 age groups (one for each year 6–17), with at least 75 boys and 75 girls in each age group. The company was able to obtain ratings from 1,922 parents with at least 80 boys and 80 girls in each of these age groups. Initial analyses of the demographic profile showed that male respondents (fathers) were slightly overrepresented in the sample (53 vs. 47% female). Ethnically White individuals were also somewhat overrepresented (74%) compared with the 2000 U.S. Census (69.1%). College-educated (bachelor's degree or higher, 42%) people were also overrepresented compared with the U.S. Census (25%). Consequently, the original sample was reduced by 6% (*N* = 122) by removing White males having bachelor's degrees or higher. Those chosen for removal were proportionately weighted across bachelor's (*N* = 62), Master's (*N* = 40), and doctoral degrees (*N* = 20) and equally distributed between male (*N* = 61) and female (*N* = 61) children so as to retain an equal representation of boys and girls at each of the original age levels. The selection of an individual for removal from among those meeting these characteristics was done at random. The final sample used to create the norms reported here therefore consisted of 1,800 parents (and their children). This slightly reduced sample is referred to henceforth as the *normative sample*. All further analyses reported in the remainder of this chapter are based on this normative sample.

Age, Sex, and Biological Relationship

The ages of the parents in the normative sample who completed the rating scale ranged from 18 to 68 years, with a mean age of 42.3 years (*SD* = 7.9). The parent respondents reported that 95.3% of the children in this survey had another parent known to them (*N* = 1,715). Those other parents ranged in age from 21 to 76 years, with a mean age of 42.5 (*SD* = 7.5). The mean age of the children in the sample was 11.8 years (*SD* = 3.7). The parent respondents were equally represented by sex: 50% fathers (*N* = 900) and 50% mothers (*N* = 900). Biological parents represented 91% of the sample. The specific breakdown of the status of the parents' biological relationships to the children follows: biological mothers, 46.43%; stepmother, 1.5%; adoptive mothers, 1.3%; foster mothers, 0.1%; biological fathers, 44.8%; stepfathers, 3.1%; adoptive fathers, 1.7%; and foster fathers = 1.1%.

Education

The breakdown in educational categories for the parent respondents in comparison with the 2000 U.S. Census (*www.census.gov*) is shown in the following:

Education category	Normative sample	U.S. Census
Less than high school	4.1%	19.1%
High school (diploma or equivalency)	28.1%	28.6%
Some college, no degree	20.6%	21.0%
Associates degree	9.2%	6.3%
Bachelor's degree	22.6%	15.5%
Graduate degree	15.4%	8.9%

The present sample is generally comparable to the U.S. population in the percentage having high school diplomas or equivalency, some college, or associate's degrees but has a slight overrepresentation of individuals with bachelor's or graduate degrees. The sample also contains a lower percentage of those having less than a high school education than appear in the U.S. Census. The breakdown of educational levels of the nonrespondent parents follows: less than high school, 6.6%; high school, 20.6%; some college, no degree, 20.6%; associate's degree, 10.2%; bachelor's degree, 22.8%; graduate degree, 14.8%. These percentages are very similar to those for the respondent parents. The mean educational level for the children in the sample was 7.4 years (*SD* = 3.5, range = kindergarten [1] to 12th grade [13]), or roughly a mid-6th-grade education.

Geographic Region

The geographic distribution of the participants was as follows in comparison with the 2000 U.S. Census:

U.S. geographic region	Normative sample	U.S. Census
Northeast	18%	19%
Midwest	28%	23%
South	31%	36%
West	23%	22%

The normative sample thus represents all regions of the United States and appears to approximate the geographic distribution of the U.S. adult population.

Ethnicity

The racial/ethnic breakdown of the normative sample is as follows relative to the 2000 U.S. Census:

Ethnic group	Normative sample	U.S. Census
White, alone	73.0%	75.1%
Black	7.7%	12.3%
Other (Asian, Native U.S.)	4.3%	6.6%
Hispanic	12.4%	12.5%
Multiracial	2.7%	2.4%

The sample contains members of all major ethnic groups in the United States and appears to approximate the racial/ethnic distribution of the United States except for a somewhat lower representation of Blacks in the normative sample relative to the U.S. Census.

Household Income

The breakdown of the normative sample by income categories is shown in the following, again relative to the 2000 U.S. Census:

Income category	Normative sample	U.S. Census
Less than $10,000	5.4%	9.5%
$10,000–$14,499	2.9%	6.3%
$15,000–$24,999	5.5%	12.8%
$25,000–$34,999	7.7%	12.8%
$35,000–$49,999	11.4%	16.5%
$50,000–$74,999	20.4%	19.5%
$75,000–$99,999	18.8%	10.2%
$100,000–$149,999	18.7%	7.7%
$150,000+	9.3%	4.6%

The mean income range was $50,000 to $59,999, whereas both the median and mode fell in the range of $60,000–$74,999. The median household income of the United States is $41,994 as of the 2000 U.S. Census. The results suggest that this sample of parents had a somewhat higher average household income than that of the entire U.S. population. However, once again these figures are not directly comparable given that the U.S. Census does not break down household income into categories such as parents with children in the age ranges used here. It is possible that parents have a somewhat higher mean household income than do individuals who are not parents in the population.

Marital Status of Parents

The marital status of the parents in the normative sample relative to the parents of children reported in the 2000 U.S. Census follows:

Marital status	Normative sample	U.S. Census
Married	81.3%	69.0%
Separated, divorced, widowed	8.3%	19.0%
Never married	4.3%	11.9%

As this table shows, the normative sample has a slightly higher representation of married parents than is the case in the U.S. population.

Employment Status of Parents

The employment status of the normative sample was: working as paid employees, 64.8%; self-employed, 8.7%; not working, on temporary layoff, 1.2%; not working, looking for work, 6.8%; retired, 1.1%; disabled, not working, 4.5%; and not working for other reasons (working as a homemaker, for instance), 12.9%. Approximately 74% of the sample was working. Comparable figures could not be located from the U.S. Census for the age range of parents and children in the normative sample. However, overall employment in the U.S. 2000 Census was 64% for individuals 18 years of age and older. The employment figure for the normative sample is similar to this figure from the 2000 U.S. Census.

To summarize the demographic characteristics, it appears that the normative sample recruited here reasonably approximates that of the U.S. adult population as based on the U.S. Census from the year 2000 concerning regional distribution, sex, race/ethnic group, and employment status. It is unclear how this sample compares with the U.S. population in household income, as such figures are not readily available from the U.S. Census for parents within this age range having children within this age range of the normative sample. The normative sample has a somewhat higher representation of parents who are married and who are college graduates.

Developmental and Psychiatric Diagnoses of Children

Parents were asked whether or not their children had ever received any of the following diagnoses from a professional. Alongside each diagnosis is the percentage of the normative sample that had received such a diagnosis:

Diagnosis	Sample
Physical disability (unable to talk or use arms unassisted)	0.3%
Language delay	5.0%
Motor skill or coordination delay	3.3%
Reading disorder or disability	4.2%
Math disorder or disability	2.4%
Spelling disorder or disability	2.4%
Writing disorder or disability	2.3%
Other academic learning disorder	1.7%
General developmental delay or mental retardation	1.2%
Tic disorder or Tourette syndrome	0.6%
Deafness or hearing disability	0.4%
Blindness or visual impairment	0.6%
Seizure disorder or epilepsy	0.8%
Attention-deficit disorder (ADD) or ADHD	9.2%
Oppositional defiant disorder	1.6%
Conduct disorder	0.3%
Any anxiety disorder	3.0%
Any depression disorder	1.8%
Bipolar disorder or manic–depression	0.8%
Autism or autistic spectrum disorder or Asperger syndrome	1.8%
Childhood schizophrenia or psychosis	0.1%
No diagnosis of any of the above	77.1%

The rates for various disorders are well within the ranges found in various epidemiological studies of the U.S. population of children (American Psychiatric Association, 2000; Mash & Barkley, 2003; see Chapter 7 also) except that children diagnosed with oppositional defiant disorder and conduct disorder appear to be underrepresented. Approximately 23% of the sample had one or more disorders. The results are reasonably consistent with research showing that on average 12–13.5% of children ages 6–12 and 16.5% of children ages 13–18 have at least one psychiatric disorder (Costello, Egger, & Angold, 2005; Roberts, Attkisson, & Rosenblatt, 1998), typically ranging between 14 and 20%, depending on methods used for diagnosis (Brandenburg, Friedman, & Silver, 1990). Some recent studies found an overall prevalence for psychiatric disorders for a 3-month period of 13.5% and lifetime prevalence throughout a 3-year follow-up during childhood of 36.7% (Costello, Mustillo, Erkanli, Keeler, & Angold, 2003). Add to the average prevalence of 13–16% the percentage having intellectual, learning, language, and motor disorders that account for another 10–12% of the population exclusive of psychiatric disorders (Boyle, Decoufle, & Yeargin-Allsop, 1994; Mash & Barkley, 2003) and one finds that on average 23–29% of the U.S. population of children have at least one developmental, learning, or psychiatric disorder. The overall prevalence of 23% in the present normative sample is therefore a close approximation of the prevalence of these disorders in the U.S. population of children.

Treatment Status of the Children

Parents were also asked to indicate whether their children had ever received any of the following types of treatment:

Treatment type	Sample
Any medication for a psychiatric or psychological disorder	8.1%
Formal tutoring outside of school for school performance	4.1%
Special education services of any type	9.4%
Speech and language therapy	11.4%
Occupational therapy	4.3%
Physical therapy	3.0%
Individual psychological counseling	9.4%
Family psychological counseling	3.9%
Group psychological therapy	0.9%
Placement in an inpatient psychiatric unit	0.7%
Attendance at a residential treatment school for children with psychological or psychiatric disorders	0.3%
None of the treatments listed above	71.6%

It is not possible to find comparable figures for the United States for all of these therapies, but a comparison with those for which figures are available suggests that these rates are reasonably similar to those found in other studies. For instance, one study using data from the National Ambulatory Medical Care Survey found a rate of psychotropic drug use of 8.3% for adolescents in 2000–2001 (Thomas, Conrad, Casler, & Goodman, 2006), a figure that had more than doubled since 1996 and one very close to that found for such drug use in our normative sample. Likewise, several studies found rates of 3.9–6.3% for children in the United States in 1996 (Olfson, Marcus, Weissman, & Jensen, 2002; Zito et al., 2003), a rate that also had more than doubled since 1987 (see Olfson et al., 2002). Given the results for the Thomas et al. (2006) study of teenagers over the subsequent term to 2001, this rate for children likely doubled again by the early 2000s (to at least 7–12%). Again, the expected rate is very similar to that found here.

Comparison of BDEFS-CA Methodology to the BRIEF

It may be useful to users of the BDEFS-CA to consider the means by which the normative sample was collected here relative to another popular rating scale used for evaluating EF in children, that being the parent form of the BRIEF. The manual for the BRIEF (Gioia et al., 2000) indicates that the vast majority of their sample was drawn only from residents of the state of Maryland, with a small community sample of adolescents (N = 18) from Cleveland, Ohio. This sample is not drawn from the entire United States. Instead, respondents came from 25 public and private schools comprising 12 elementary, 9 middle, and 4 high schools. Therefore, age groups are not equally represented in this sample, given the oversampling of younger grades and hence age groups. In contrast, the normative sample for the BDEFS-CA was drawn from all nine major regions of the United States, with equal representation at all 12 age levels and without using schools as a mediator for data collection. Moreover, the parent respondents for the BRIEF were largely mothers (83.2%), and the sample featured an overrepresentation of Whites (80% vs. 69% of the U.S. 2000 Census) and a corresponding underrepresentation of Hispanics (3% vs. 12.5% of the U.S. 2000 Census). The normative sample for the BDEFS-CA has an equal representation of fathers and mothers and a much closer representation of ethnic Whites (73%) and Hispanics (12.4%) to the U.S. population.

Other differences between the BDEFS-CA and the BRIEF are overall sample size, gender representation, and scale construction. The BRIEF normative sample included 1,419 children comprising 604 boys and 815 girls, suggesting that boys may be underrepresented in this sample in comparison with the general population. The BDEFS-CA used a larger sample of 1,800 parents who reported on equal numbers of male and female children (900 each). Generally, larger samples can be expected to be more representative of the population of interest. Also, the BRIEF items were assigned to their respective subscales initially based on their face validity—the apparent similarity of their content. Eight subscales were created by this method, making it appear as if the scale is evaluating eight different EF components. But this is not an empirically based approach. When all of these items were factor analyzed, the results showed that the scale consists of just two empirically derived dimensions—one reflecting behavioral inhibition (and emotion regulation) and the other reflecting metacognition (working memory, time management, organization, problem solving, etc.) (Gioia et al., 2000). The BDEFS-CA, instead, began with a large sample of items constructed to represent the most commonly described EF components. An empirical approach was then used to assign items to scales based on the results of factor analyses of multiple samples of adults across the human lifespan (ages 18–92 years) and then on an analysis of a representative sample of U.S. children as reported in this manual. Five factors or dimensions of EF were obtained and replicated across the adult and child normative samples, instead of just the two represented in the BRIEF.

Another important issue has to do with filtering of the normative sample. Children included in the BRIEF normative sample could not have a history of special education or be on psychotropic medication. However, as noted earlier, a substantial minority of the U.S. child population qualifies for a psychological or educational disorder that could make them eligible for special education services or for psychotropic medication (usually cited as 20–25%). Indeed, children receiving special education reflect a wide range of developmental, learning, behavioral, and psychiatric disorders. Such children would be expected to have some of the highest scores on a rating scale of executive deficits. Filtering out such a sizeable minority of children can result in a normative sample that is not representative of the U.S. population of children and compresses the upper end of the distribution of executive deficit symptoms. Comparison of any ratings of a child patient with such a sample would make it far more likely that the individual's scores might deviate significantly (clinically) from this supernormal sample than from one based on a representative sample of the general U.S. population of children having a proportionate representation of various disorders or history of treatment, as was done here.

The point is not merely academic. The mean of the EF Summary Score on the BDEFS-CA for the normative sample is 113 with a standard deviation (*SD*) of 40. If all children receiving psychotropic medication or having a history of special education are removed, the mean becomes 106 (*SD* = 34), clearly showing the leftward compression of the distribution. Consider as well that a child obtaining an EF Summary Score of 162 on the BDEFS-CA would place at the 88th percentile, which would be considered at the higher end of the normal range but not an indication of clinical deficiency. That same score would be at the 93rd percentile if all children receiving medication or who had received special education were removed from the sample. It would now be viewed as evidence of clinically significant deficiency in EF. This creates a tendency to overidentify children as having clinically significant EF deficits. To answer the question concerning a person's relative position within the general population requires comparison with a representative sample of that entire child and adolescent population rather than a comparison of relative position with a sample characterized only by nondisordered individuals. Children in the BDEFS-CA normative sample were not screened out because of any psychiatric or educational condition or for using a psychotropic medication; instead, efforts were made to obtain as representative a sample of U.S. children and adolescents as possible.

One final difference between the scales is the cost of use extended over time. The BRIEF materials are more expensive to purchase initially, and it also requires additional answer sheets to be repeatedly purchased over time as the need arises. In contrast, the BDEFS-CA comes with limited permission for the purchaser to photocopy the scale for use in his/her clinical practice with no need to continually repurchase additional answer forms and scoring profiles, thus saving the owner considerable time, labor, and expense, especially over extended use of the scale.

The results of the factor analyses of the scale and construction of the individual subscales based on this normative sample are discussed in the next chapter.

CHAPTER 4

Factor Analysis, Scale Construction, and Item Frequencies

This chapter discusses the results of the factor analyses used to uncover the underlying dimensions of EF in the daily life activities of children and adolescents as reported by their parents on the BDEFS-CA. It then discusses the use of those results to construct the final version and subscales of the BDEFS-CA. Thereafter, the frequencies with which the items were endorsed by the normative sample are presented and discussed.

Factor Analysis

As indicated in Chapter 2, the BDEFS-CA represents a downward extension of the BDEFS for adults. The highest 14 items loading on each of the five factors of the BDEFS were chosen for inclusion in this parent version. The results of the factor analysis for the adult form (Barkley, 2011a) revealed five factors: Self-Management to Time, Self-Organization/Problem Solving, Self-Restraint (Inhibition), Self-Motivation, and Self-Regulation of Emotion.

Using the original and entire sample of 1,922 children, the ratings on the 70-item BDEFS-CA were submitted to a principal-components factor analysis (PCFA). The initial results prior to rotation revealed five factors that had eigenvalues greater than 1 that accounted for 68.5% of the variance. These unrotated factors were as follows:

- Factor 1: Eigenvalue = 37.07, variance = 52.96%
- Factor 2: Eigenvalue = 4.31, variance = 6.15%
- Factor 3: Eigenvalue = 3.51, variance = 5.02%
- Factor 4: Eigenvalue = 1.60, variance = 2.29%
- Factor 5: Eigenvalue = 1.48, variance = 2.12%

Inspection of the initial factor structure showed that all items had their highest loadings in a positive direction on Factor 1, making this a unitary executive dysfunction factor. Because EF is viewed here as reflecting self-regulation (see Chapter 1), this factor can be viewed as one representing deficient self-regulation. The finding of a large general factor in the initial PCFA is consistent with earlier research, discussed in Chapter 1, that suggests that EF is a unitary construct, at least at this initial broad level of analysis. It is also consistent with earlier research on the prototype of the adult BDEFS (Biederman, Petty, Fried, Doyle, et al., 2008; Fedele, Hartung, Canu, & Wilkowski, 2010). Yet the smaller factors also explained another 15.5% of the variance. Their existence implies that EF can also be viewed as somewhat diverse in its composition. Factor 2 had its highest loadings in a negative direction. Those items came from the original Self-Regulation of Emotion factor, and a few were related to Self-Restraint, which were mainly the two emotion items on that scale. Factor 3 had its highest loadings on items related to Self-Organization/Problem Solving. Factor 4 had its highest loadings, again in a negative direction, on those items evaluating Self-Restraint (Inhibition). And the last factor had its highest loadings in a positive direction on items evaluating Self-Management to Time. These results replicated those found for the PCFA for the adult scale prior to rotation.

The parent ratings were submitted initially to a varimax rotation, designed to maximize as many values in each column of the factor-loading coefficient table as close to zero as possible. This approach is typically used in an attempt to reduce the degree of correlation among the items (variables). But the ratings were also submitted to a promax rotation, which is frequently used when variables are known to be correlated, as are the EF items. That rotation allows items to be correlated with more than one factor. Both approaches yielded the same eventual factor structure. The results of the PCFA are shown in Table 4.1. It reports the factor loadings for both the varimax and promax rotations.

The first factor was labeled Self-Regulation of Emotion, identical to its label on the adult version of this scale. It contained 16 items, had an eigenvalue of 12.93 after rotation, and explained 18.5% of the variance after rotation. The seven highest loading items are shown next, in descending order to give the reader some idea about the conceptual content of this dimension:

- Not able to be reasonable once he/she is emotional
- Cannot seem to distract him/herself away from whatever is upsetting him/her emotionally to help calm down. Can't refocus his/her mind to a more positive framework
- Has trouble calming him/herself down once he/she is emotionally upset
- Not able to rechannel or redirect his/her emotions

(text resumes on page 44)

TABLE 4.1. Rotated Factor Loadings for BDEFS-CA Items Based on PCFA with Varimax (and Promax) Rotations

	Factors				
Factor name/scale items[a]	1	2	3	4	5
1. Self-Regulation of Emotion					
EF41. Has a low tolerance for frustrating situations	.576 (.748)				
EF42. Cannot inhibit his/her emotions	.626 (.795)				
EF57. Quick to get angry or become upset	.667 (.813)				
EF58. Overreact emotionally	.702 (.823)				
EF59. Easily excitable	.570 (.746)				
EF60. Not able to inhibit showing strong negative or positive emotions	.635 (.797)				
EF61. Has trouble calming him/herself down once he/she is emotionally upset	.807 (.862)				
EF62. Not able to be reasonable once he/she is emotional	.813 (.882)				
EF63. Cannot seem to distract him/herself away from whatever is upsetting them emotionally to help calm down. Can't refocus his/her mind to a more positive framework.	.812 (.892)				
EF64. Not able to manage his/her emotions in order to accomplish his/her goals successfully or get along well with others	.766 (.879)				
EF65. Remain emotional or upset longer than other children	.739 (.830)				
EF66. Find it difficult to walk away from emotionally upsetting encounters with others or leave situations in which he/she have become very emotional	.777 (.853)				
EF67. Not able to rechannel or redirect his/her emotions into more positive ways or outlets when he/she gets upset	.794 (.894)				
EF68. Not able to evaluate an emotionally upsetting event more objectively or reasonably	.778 (.886)				
EF69. Not able to reevaluate or redefine negative events into a more positive viewpoint when he/she feels strong emotions	.761 (.873)				
EF70. Emotionally impulsive or quick to show or express his/her feelings	.687 (.826)				
2. Self-Organization/Problem-Solving					
EF15. When shown something complicated to do, he/she cannot keep it in mind so as to do it correctly		.549 (.730)			
EF16. Has trouble considering various ways of doing things		.584 (.750)			

(cont.)

TABLE 4.1. *(cont.)*

Factor name/scale items[a]	Factors 1	2	3	4	5
EF17. Has difficulty saying what he/she wants to say		.734 (.792)			
EF18. Unable to come up with or invent as many solutions to problems as others		.713 (.818)			
EF19. At a loss for words when he/she wants to explain something		.739 (.799)			
EF20. Has trouble explaining his/her ideas as well or as quickly as others		.803 (.863)			
EF21. Not as creative or inventive as others of his/her age		.638 (.679)			
EF22. Has trouble learning new or complex activities		.689 (.785)			
EF23. Has difficulty explaining things in his/her proper order or sequence		.746 (.833)			
EF24. Can't seem to get to the point of his/her explanations		.739 (.819)			
EF25. Has trouble doing things in his/her proper order or sequence		.708 (.834)			
EF26. Unable to "think on his/her feet," problem-solve, or respond effectively to unexpected events		.697 (.806)			
EF27. Slow at solving problems he/she encounters in his/her daily life		.687 (.818)			
EF28. Doesn't seem to process information quickly or accurately		.756 (.844)			
3. Self-Management to Time					
EF1. Procrastinates or puts off doing things until the last minute			.716 (.768)		
EF2. Has a poor sense of time			.719 (.812)		
EF3. Wastes or doesn't manage his/her time well			.759 (.846)		
EF4. Not prepared on time for schoolwork or assigned tasks given at home			.636 (.770)		
EF5. Has trouble planning ahead or preparing for upcoming events			.683 (.822)		
EF6. Can't seem to accomplish the goals he/she sets for him/herself			.535 (.746)		
EF7. Not able to get things done unless there is an immediate deadline or consequence			.669 (.812)		

(cont.)

TABLE 4.1. *(cont.)*

Factor name/scale items[a]	Factors 1	2	3	4	5
EF8. Has difficulty judging how much time it will take to do something or get somewhere			.672 (.801)		
EF9. Has trouble starting the work he/she is asked to do			.649 (.808)		
EF10. Has difficulty sticking with his/her work and getting it done			.617 (808)		
EF11. Not able to prepare in advance for things he/she knows he/she is supposed to do			.642 (.817)		
EF12. Has trouble following through on what he/she agrees to do			.593 (.805)		
EF14. Has difficulty doing the work he/she is asked to do in the order of its priority or importance; can't "prioritize" well			.569 (.795)		
4. Self-Motivation					
EF43. Takes short cuts in his/her chores, schoolwork, or other assignments and does not do all that he/she is supposed to do				.615 (.820)	
EF44. Quits working if his/her chores, schoolwork, or other assignments are boring for him/her to do				.589 (.822)	
EF45. Does not put much effort into his/her chores, schoolwork, or other assignments				.680 (.874)	
EF46. Seems lazy or unmotivated				.612 (.780)	
EF47. Has to depend on other people to help get his/her chores, schoolwork, or other assignments done				.608 (.826)	
EF48. Things must have an immediate payoff for him/her or he/she is not able to get them done				.577 (.819)	
EF49. Has difficulty resisting the urge to do something fun or more interesting when he/she is supposed to be working				.520 (.790)	
EF50. Inconsistent in the quality or quantity of his/her work performance				.625 (.854)	
EF51. Unable to work without supervision or frequent instruction				.550 (.803)	
EF52. Lacks willpower or self-determination				.583 (.828)	
EF53. Not able to work toward longer-term or delayed rewards				.580 (.840)	
EF54. Not able to resist doing things that produce immediate rewards even if it is not good for him/her in the long run				.483 (.782)	

(cont.)

TABLE 4.1. *(cont.)*

	Factors				
Factor name/scale items[a]	1	2	3	4	5
EF55. Gives up too easily if something requires much effort				.567 (.822)	
EF56. Not able to get started on his/her chores, school projects, or work without a lot of prodding or encouragement from others				.536 (.808)	
5. Self-Restraint (Inhibition)					
EF13. Has trouble with self-discipline (self-control)					.448 (.767)
EF29. Has difficulty waiting for things; has to have things or do things he/she wants right away					.491 (.741)
EF30. Makes decisions impulsively					.588 (.795)
EF31. Unable to inhibit his/her reactions to events or to what others say or do to him/her; reacts on impulse					.568 (.815)
EF32. Has difficulty stopping what he/she is doing when it is time to do so					.500 (.737)
EF33. Has difficulty correcting his/her behavior when he/she is given feedback about his/her mistakes					.478 (.797)
EF34. Makes impulsive comments					.630 (.832)
EF35. Likely to do things without considering the consequences for doing them					.669 (.888)
EF36. Acts without thinking things over					.650 (.877)
EF37. Finds it hard to take another person's perspective about a problem or situation					.491 (.774)
EF38. Doesn't stop and talk things over with him/herself before deciding to do something					.613 (.856)
EF39. Has trouble following the rules in a situation					.568 (.814)
EF40. Engages in risky behavior or risk taking					.550 (.715)

[a]The number beginning with EF in front of each item reflects the order in which this item appeared on the scale as it was given to the normative sample.

- Finds it difficult to walk away from his/her emotionally upsetting encounters with others or leave situations in which he/she has become very emotional
- Not able to manage his/her emotions in order to accomplish his/her goals successfully or get along well with others
- Remains emotional or upset longer than other children

The items were generated originally using Gross's modal model of emotion and its self-regulation (Gross, 1998; Gross & John, 2003; Gross & Thompson, 2007). The results here show the same high level of consistency with this model as did the adult scale (Barkley, 2011a) and clearly support the labeling of this scale as one involving deficits in the self-regulation of emotions.

The second factor had an eigenvalue of 10.45 after rotation, accounted for 14.9% of the variance after rotation, and contained the same 14 items that were found on the Self-Organization/Problem Solving subscale of the adult form. And so the same label was retained for this factor. Others have referred to this dimension as one of cognitive inflexibility with regard to the prototype for the adult BDEFS (Fedele et al., 2010). But in the initial research with that prototype of the scale (Barkley & Murphy, 2011), this factor was given the name Self-Organization/Problem Solving, and so that name is retained here, as well as in the final version of the BDEFS adult form, for consistency. The seven highest loading items, again in descending order, were:

- Has trouble explaining his/her ideas as well or as quickly as others
- Doesn't seem to process information quickly or accurately
- Has difficulty explaining things in his/her proper order or sequence
- At a loss for words when he/she wants to explain something
- Can't seem to get to the point of his/her explanations
- Has difficulty saying what he/she wants to say
- Unable to come up with or invent as many solutions to problems as others

Factor 3 had an eigenvalue of 9.72. It accounted for 13.9% of the variance after rotation and comprised 13 of the 14 items from the adult scale that reflected Self-Management to Time. Some might consider this a time-management factor. Technically, however, one does not manage time but oneself relative to the passage of time, which flows at a constant rate regardless of one's efforts to manage his/her actions relative to it. It is the sensing of time and one's self-management to it that is apparently the essence of this factor. Others have referred to this dimension as a failure to plan and persist in reference to the prototype of the BDEFS (Fedele et al., 2010). But it was called Self-Management to Time on the original prototype of the adult scale (Barkley & Murphy, 2011) and on the eventual published BDEFS (Barkley, 2011a), so it retains that name here. As noted before, the 14th item from this scale loaded slightly more highly on the Self-Restraint scale and so was placed on that factor in the BDEFS-CA. The seven highest loading items on this factor in descending order were:

- Wastes or doesn't manage his/her time well
- Has a poor sense of time
- Procrastinates or puts off doing things until the last minute

- Has trouble planning ahead or preparing for upcoming events
- Has difficulty judging how much time it will take to do something or get somewhere
- Not able to get things done unless there is an immediate deadline or consequence
- Has trouble starting the work he/she is asked to do

The fourth factor had an eigenvalue of 7.76, contained 14 items, and was labeled the same as on the adult version of the scale (Barkley, 2011a): Self-Motivation. This factor accounted for 11.1% of the variance after rotation. It clearly reflects the construct of motivation and has been so labeled by others using the prototype of the adult BDEFS (Barkley & Murphy, 2011; Fedele et al., 2010). The seven highest loading items on this factor in descending order were:

- Does not put much effort into his/her chores, schoolwork, or other assignments
- Inconsistent in the quality or quantity of his/her work performance
- Takes shortcuts in his/her chores, schoolwork, or other assignments and does not do all that he/she is supposed to do
- Seems lazy or unmotivated
- Has to depend on other people to help get his/her chores, schoolwork, or other assignments done
- Quits working if his/her chores, schoolwork, or other assignments are boring for him/her to do
- Lacks willpower or self-determination

Finally, Factor 5 had an eigenvalue of 7.13 after rotation. This factor accounted for 10.2% of the variance after rotation. It replicated the same factor found on the prototype (Barkley & Murphy, 2011; Fedele et al., 2010) and final versions (Barkley, 2011a) of the adult BDEFS scale and so was similarly labeled as Self-Restraint (Inhibition). It contained 13 items, 12 of which loaded on this same dimension on the adult form. The third item migrated over from the original Self-Management to Time factor and dealt with a lack of self-control or self-discipline. The items on this scale reflect impulsive thought and action, or disinhibition (Fedele et al., 2010). It clearly reflects a lack of self-restraint and is so named in keeping with the view that EF reflects self-regulation (see Chapter 1). The seven highest loading items in descending order were:

- Likely to do things without considering the consequences for doing them
- Acts without thinking things over
- Makes impulsive comments
- Doesn't stop and talk things over with him/herself before deciding to do something
- Makes decisions impulsively
- Unable to inhibit his/her reactions to events or to what others say or do to him/her; reacts on impulse
- Has trouble following the rules in a situation

Scale Construction

The items in Table 4.1 were used to create the subscales for the BDEFS-CA published here. All but three items were kept in their original sequence on the scale just as they were presented to the normative sample during the survey. That order is shown in the table by the number in front of each item. Item arrangement or organization on a scale such as this can influence symptom endorsements by respondents (Mitchell, Knouse, Nelson-Gray, & Kwapil, 2009). And so items need to be arranged as close to their original sequence in the norming process as possible so as not to reduce the applicability of the norms for the final version of the scale. Three items, however, had to be moved from that original sequence because the results of the previous PCFA showed that, for children, they should actually be assigned to different factors than was originally thought to be the case based on the normative data for the adult scale (Barkley, 2011a). These relocations were discussed earlier and are reflected in Table 4.1 as the numbers that appear out of sequence (nos. 13, 41, and 42). The items were therefore slightly reorganized into their new positions so that all items pertaining to a single factor were located in the same section of the scale, just as they were presented to the normative sample, except for the three items just discussed. Items were then renumbered sequentially to create the final version of the scale as it appears in the Appendix (not as it appears in Table 4.1). Because the items for Self-Management to Time appeared first in this sequence, they were kept in that order, followed by the items for Self-Organization/Problem Solving, then the items for Self-Restraint, followed by the items for Self-Motivation, and concluding with the section containing the items for the Self-Regulation of Emotion. Therefore, five subscale sections exist on the BDEFS-CA. This method or organization of items on the scale retains the sequence and organization as near as possible to the manner in which it was given to the normative sample. It also permits ease of scoring the scale, as the examiner can simply sum the scores for the items in each section (subscale) to compute that scale's score. These section or subscale total raw scores can then be summed to compute the EF Summary Score (see Chapter 9 for detailed scoring instructions).

Creation of the ADHD-EF Index

Previous research using both the prototype of the BDEFS (Barkley & Murphy, 2011) and its final version (Barkley, 2011a) indicated that adult ADHD is associated with significant impairment in EF in daily life activities in the majority of adults with the disorder. The same has been found for children with ADHD in studies using the BRIEF, another rating scale discussed in the last chapter for assessing EF deficits in children (Gioia et al., 2000; Mares, McLuckie, Schwartz, & Saini, 2007; Reddy, Hale, & Brodzinsky, 2011). The parents in this project were provided with a rating scale containing the 18 DSM-IV ADHD items and, if they had answered any item as occurring "Often or more frequently," they were given questions concerning impairment in home, school, social, and community domains. All items were rated the same as those on the BDEFS-CA. This ADHD scale was completed at the same time as the BDEFS-CA. The results of this scale were used to select those children who placed at or above the 93rd percentile, or approximately 1.5 *SD* above the mean in their total raw scores on this scale. Although a score of 41 fell at +1.5 *SD*, a score of 43 represented the actual 93rd percentile given the skewed distribution of scores typical of such ratings. For this purpose, a score of 43 or higher was therefore used to place a child within this significantly elevated range of symptoms. Of the original full sample of 1,922, 142 children met this threshold and were classified as being the probable ADHD group. An impairment requirement was then imposed on this subset of cases by which the parent had to indicate whether the child was impaired in home, school, or social relationships. There were 125 children who had elevated ADHD symptoms (≥ 93rd percentile) and also were reported as impaired in one or more of these domains. These cases were then classified as having probable ADHD with impairment according to these research criteria.

Binary logistic regression with forward conditional entry was then used to identify the best EF items for discriminating this group from the rest of the sample. The results showed that 10 items were needed to achieve the best classification of 97% overall accuracy (70% of ADHD cases and 99% of controls). These were items 5, 21, 22, 24, 28, 36, 49, 53, 59, and 68, as shown in Table 4.1. These 10 symptoms (and their factor assignments) were:

- Has trouble planning ahead or preparing for upcoming events (Self-Management to Time)
- Not as creative or inventive as others of his/her age (Self-Organization)
- Has trouble learning new or complex activities (Self-Organization)
- Can't seem to get to the point of his/her explanations (Self-Organization)
- Doesn't seem to process information quickly or accurately (Self-Organization)
- Acts without thinking things over (Self-Restraint)
- Has difficulty resisting the urge to do something fun or more interesting when he/she is supposed to be working (Self-Motivation)
- Not able to work toward longer-term or delayed rewards (Self-Motivation)
- Easily excitable (Self-Regulation of Emotion)
- Not able to evaluate an emotionally upsetting event more objectively or reasonably (Self-Regulation of Emotion)

Although information was available on the percentage of children in the sample who had received a professional's diagnosis of ADHD or ADD according to parents (see previous discussion), this diagnosis was not used here as a means of classifying children as having ADHD for purposes of finding the best set of EF items to identify ADHD. Relying on parental reports of a professional diagnosis of ADHD was believed to be much less rigorous than the empirical research criteria used earlier for several reasons. First, 53% of the children who had levels of ADHD symptoms sufficient to place in the top 7% of this sample did not actually have a professional diagnosis of ADHD. And just 44% of those having such a professional diagnosis placed at this level of severity of ADHD symptoms. Second, it is unclear what criteria professionals may have used to render a diagnosis of ADHD given that the children in this sample were classified based purely on parental reports that the children had received such a diagnosis. Third, the professional diagnosis included not just ADHD but also ADD. That diagnostic term is often used currently in clinical practice to refer to children who may have the predominantly inattentive type of ADHD. But many of those children have been found to have symptoms of sluggish cognitive tempo (SCT), which may not be a subtype of ADHD at all but a separate attention disorder (Barkley, in press; Milich, Ballentine, & Lynam, 2001). Those cases are characterized as being "daydreamy," staring, spacey, mentally confused and foggy, lethargic, and hypoactive, among other symptoms. If that is even partially the case in this sample of ADHD/ADD cases, then very different symptoms of EF may be needed to identify that subset of individuals clinically diagnosed as having ADD than would be the case for those with ADHD. The issue cannot be examined here because the question presented to parents was whether or not their child had received a diagnosis of ADHD or ADD, with no distinction being made in that item between the diagnoses. Thus the empirical research criteria for ADHD as developed here were preferred as the best approach to identifying cases having probable ADHD.

Based on this analysis, the 10 items from the BDEFS-CA that were best at distinguishing the empirically defined ADHD cases discussed earlier were used to create an ADHD-EF Index score. That score can be used to guide clinicians in identifying children who may be at high risk of qualifying for a diagnosis of ADHD. These items can be scored separately on the BDEFS-CA for just this purpose. Norms are provided on the EF Profiles in the Appendix to do this separately from scoring each of the five EF factors or dimensions of the scale.

Creation of the BDEFS-CA Short Form

There may be situations in which the examiner or parent does not have time to complete the full long form of the BDEFS-CA (70 items) and desires a quick screening tool to assess the possibility that deficits in EF in daily life may exist in a particular child. The BDEFS-CA Short Form was created to serve this purpose. It is composed of the four highest loading items from each of the five subscales and provides a 20-item EF screener. The BDEFS-CA Short Form can be found in the Appendix, along with the 70-item Long Form and EF Profiles. A separate EF Profile score sheet was created just for this short form apart from those used to score the full BDEFS-CA Long Form. Information on the reliability and validity of both the long and short forms is provided in later chapters.

Frequency of Item Responses

It is clinically and scientifically informative to examine the percentage of parents in the normative sample (N = 1,800) who endorsed each of the responses for each item. This gives an indication of how common or uncommon such symptoms of EF deficits in daily life activities are likely to be in children and adolescents. This information can also be used to determine how frequently each item should occur to indicate that this item at that frequency level can be judged to be a "symptom" or actual deficit rather than a common occurrence in the population. For instance, if an item is answered by the vast majority of parents with an answer of "rarely" or "sometimes," then responses of "often" or "very often" can be considered to be indicative of a symptom of an EF deficit for a child. A symptom in this case would be a behavioral complaint that occurs at a frequency that is relatively low in the population and so may be indicative of disorder. Whether it is or not, of course, is eventually a question of validity. It should be tested against other forms of information, particularly that dealing with impairment.

To gain some idea about how often parents endorse items of EF problems in their child's daily life, the percentage of parents in the original full sample who endorsed each of the possible answers to each item was computed. The results appear in Table 4.2. This is interesting information for neuropsychologists, developmental psychologists, and others who may have an interest in knowing the proportion of the population that endorses particular types of EF symptoms at various relative frequency estimates. What this table clearly shows is that for the vast majority of items, with a few exceptions, most of a general population sample of parents endorses most items at a frequency of either "never or rarely" or "sometimes." Answers of "often" or "very often" appeared to occur in most cases in less than 11% of the population and in the majority of cases less than 5% (though clearly there are a few exceptions). So if one wanted to identify a symptom of EF, it does not seem at all unreasonable to use an answer of "often" or "very often" to indicate the possibility of symptom status. The examiner should therefore focus not just on scoring the BDEFS-CA through simple summation of items but should inspect the scale for items on each subscale that were endorsed with responses of 3 (*Often*) or 4 (*Very often*). Doing this can provide another perspective on just how symptomatic a child may be in each component of EF assessed by each subscale.

Creation of the Scores from the Scale

As discussed previously, using the item loadings shown in Table 4.1, items were grouped on the scale in sections representing their respective factors, and the item sequences then were renumbered sequentially. The sections of the scale were then organized in the same sequence in which they had been presented to the normative sample. Thirteen items were assigned to the Self-Management to Time factor subscale constituting Section 1 of the scale. There were 14 items on the Self-Organization/Problem Solving factor scale (Section 2), 13 on the Self-Restraint factor scale (Section 3), 14 on the Self-Motivation factor scale (Section 4), and 16 on the Self-Regulation of Emotions factor scale (Section 5). These made up the BDEFS-CA Long Form. Items within each factor scale (subscale) were then summed to create the raw score for that subscale. The five subscale scores were then summed as well to create an EF Summary Score. Two additional scores were created besides these six scores. The first was the ADHD-EF Index, consisting of the sum of the 10 items that were found to be the optimal items for classifying children in the normative sample who had probable ADHD with impairment. The second was an EF Symptom Count, which consisted of a frequency count of the number of items

(text resumes on page 53)

TABLE 4.2. Percentage of the Normative Sample (N = 1,800) That Endorsed Each Possible Answer to Each Item on the BDEFS-CA

		Never or rarely	Sometimes	Often	Very often
1. Self-Management to Time items					
EF1.	Procrastinates or puts off doing things until the last minute	19.8	46.7	21.8	11.7
EF2.	Has a poor sense of time	39.1	39.8	14.4	6.7
EF3.	Wastes or doesn't manage his/her time well	26.8	47.3	18.1	7.7
EF4.	Not prepared on time for schoolwork or assigned tasks given at home	50.8	33.6	10.6	5.1
EF5.	Has trouble planning ahead or preparing for upcoming events	46.8	38.1	11.4	3.7
EF6.	Can't seem to accomplish the goals he/she sets for him/herself	60.3	31.3	5.8	2.6
EF7.	Not able to get things done unless there is an immediate deadline or consequence	40.8	38.8	14.9	5.6
EF8.	Has difficulty judging how much time it will take to do something or get somewhere	39.9	42.9	11.9	5.3
EF9.	Has trouble starting the work he/she is asked to do	40.7	38.8	14.5	6.0
EF10.	Has difficulty sticking with his/her work and getting it done	45.7	36.2	12.2	5.9
EF11.	Not able to prepare in advance for things he/she knows he/she is supposed to do	45.3	41.2	9.2	4.2
EF12.	Has trouble following through on what he/she agrees to do	45.6	39.6	10.2	4.6
EF13.	Has trouble with self-discipline (self-control)	50.4	34.5	9.0	6.1
EF14.	Has difficulty doing the work he/she is asked to do in the order of its priority or importance; can't "prioritize" well	46.3	37.7	11.2	4.8
2. Self-Organization/Problem Solving items					
EF15.	When shown something complicated to do, he/she cannot keep it in mind so as to do it correctly	59.7	29.9	6.8	3.6
EF16.	Has trouble considering various ways of doing things	55.1	34.4	7.7	2.7
EF17.	Has difficulty saying what he/she wants to say	67.7	24.5	5.6	2.3
EF18.	Unable to come up with or invent as many solutions to problems as others	65.9	26.6	5.4	2.2
EF19.	At a loss for words when he/she wants to explain something	67.9	25.0	4.7	2.3
EF20.	Has trouble explaining his/her ideas as well or as quickly as others	68.8	23.4	4.9	2.9
EF21.	Not as creative or inventive as others of his/her age	80.4	15.9	2.3	1.3
EF22.	Has trouble learning new or complex activities	71.6	22.7	3.9	1.7
EF23.	Has difficulty explaining things in his/her proper order or sequence	74.9	19.6	3.8	1.7
EF24.	Can't seem to get to the point of his/her explanations	69.4	23.3	4.9	2.3
EF25.	Has trouble doing things in his/her proper order or sequence	73.4	21.8	3.1	1.7

(cont.)

TABLE 4.2. *(cont.)*

	Never or rarely	Sometimes	Often	Very often
EF26. Unable to "think on his/her feet," problem-solve, or respond effectively to unexpected events	63.7	29.8	4.4	2.1
EF27. Slow at solving problems he/she encounters in his/her daily life	69.7	24.9	3.9	1.6
EF28. Doesn't seem to process information quickly or accurately	74.8	19.4	3.7	2.1
3. Self-Restraint (Inhibition) items				
EF29. Has difficulty waiting for things; has to have things or do things he/she wants right away	51.7	30.8	11.4	6.1
EF30. Makes decisions impulsively	43.6	41.9	9.6	4.9
EF31. Unable to inhibit his/her reactions to events or to what others say or do to him/her; reacts on impulse	55.1	32.0	8.8	4.1
EF32. Has difficulty stopping what he/she is doing when it is time to do so	50.1	36.8	9.2	3.9
EF33. Has difficulty correcting his/her behavior when he/she is given feedback about his/her mistakes	56.3	32.1	7.6	4.0
EF34. Makes impulsive comments	49.1	35.5	9.7	5.7
EF35. Likely to do things without considering the consequences for doing them	50.1	36.1	8.3	5.6
EF36. Acts without thinking things over	43.4	42.8	8.7	5.1
EF37. Finds it hard to take another person's perspective about a problem or situation	50.4	36.6	8.9	4.1
EF38. Doesn't stop and talk things over with him/herself before deciding to do something	52.4	36.4	7.4	3.8
EF39. Has trouble following the rules in a situation	66.8	25.1	4.8	3.3
EF40. Engages in risky behavior or risk taking	75.8	17.7	3.8	2.7
EF41. Has a low tolerance for frustrating situations	37.7	43.1	13.3	5.9
EF42. Cannot inhibit his/her emotions	52.5	34.8	8.6	4.2
4. Self-Motivation items				
EF43. Takes short cuts in his/her chores, schoolwork, or other assignments and does not do all that he/she is supposed to do	45.1	37.0	11.2	6.7
EF44. Quits working if his/her chores, schoolwork, or other assignments are boring for them to do	49.2	34.4	9.9	6.4
EF45. Does not put much effort into his/her chores, schoolwork, or other assignments	51.4	33.3	9.2	6.1
EF46. Seems lazy or unmotivated	51.8	34.8	8.4	5.0
EF47. Has to depend on other people to help get his/her chores, schoolwork, or other assignments done	60.6	28.5	6.7	4.2
EF48. Things must have an immediate payoff for him/her or he/she is not able to get them done	59.2	28.3	8.6	3.9

(cont.)

TABLE 4.2. *(cont.)*

	Never or rarely	Sometimes	Often	Very often
EF49. Has difficulty resisting the urge to do something fun or more interesting when he/she is supposed to be working	39.9	40.2	12.9	7.1
EF50. Inconsistent in the quality or quantity of his/her work performance	57.7	30.3	6.9	5.1
EF51. Unable to work without supervision or frequent instruction	58.1	29.8	7.7	4.5
EF52. Lacks willpower or self-determination	61.1	29.4	6.0	3.5
EF53. Not able to work toward longer-term or delayed rewards	59.3	29.7	7.8	3.2
EF54. Not able to resist doing things that produce immediate rewards even if it is not good for him/her in the long run	59.4	30.5	7.0	3.1
EF55. Gives up too easily if something requires much effort	46.2	38.7	9.9	5.2
EF56. Not able to get started on his/her chores, school projects, or work without a lot of prodding or encouragement from others	45.2	36.9	11.3	6.6
5. Self-Regulation of Emotion items				
EF57. Quick to get angry or become upset	49.3	33.4	10.4	6.8
EF58. Overreacts emotionally	45.3	36.6	10.7	7.4
EF59. Easily excitable	51.5	32.5	10.2	5.8
EF60. Not able to inhibit showing strong negative or positive emotions	59.6	28.6	7.7	4.1
EF61. Has trouble calming him/herself down once he/she is emotionally upset	55.8	31.5	8.3	4.3
EF62. Not able to be reasonable once he/she is emotional	55.0	30.6	10.2	4.2
EF63. Cannot seem to distract him/herself away from whatever is upsetting him/her emotionally to help calm down. Can't refocus his/her mind to a more positive framework.	60.7	28.3	7.8	3.3
EF64. Not able to manage his/her emotions in order to accomplish his/her goals successfully or get along well with others	69.1	22.4	5.5	3.0
EF65. Remains emotional or upset longer than other children	74.9	17.2	5.2	2.7
EF66. Finds it difficult to walk away from emotionally upsetting encounters with others or leave situations in which he/she has become very emotional	67.7	23.7	5.3	3.4
EF67. Not able to rechannel or redirect his/her emotions into more positive ways or outlets when he/she gets upset	62.4	27.8	6.6	3.2
EF68. Not able to evaluate an emotionally upsetting event more objectively or reasonably	62.0	27.2	7.3	3.5
EF69. Not able to reevaluate or redefine negative events into a more positive viewpoint when he/she feels strong emotions	61.4	28.8	6.6	3.2
EF70. Emotionally impulsive or quick to show or express his/her feelings	53.2	31.2	10.3	5.3

Note. Items are arranged in the order in which they appeared in the scale given to parents, not in the final published version of the scale in the Appendix.

that were answered 3 (*Often*) or 4 (*Very Often*) across the entire 70-item scale. Thus eight scores can be computed from the long form of the BDEFS-CA.

Then two scores were created for the BDEFS-CA Short Form (20 items). The first was the EF Summary Score, representing the sum of all 20 items on this scale. The second was the EF Symptom Count, representing the total number of these 20 items that were answered with a 3 (*Often*) or 4 (*Very Often*). Separate scores for each of the five subscales were not created for the short form as only four items from each factor-based subscale are represented on this form, a number believed to be far too small for such purposes.

The next chapter describes the relationship of these various BDEFS-CA scores to the demographic and other factors associated with the normative sample of 1,800 parents. These issues pertain to the question of how best to present the norms provided in this manual for purposes of scoring of the long and short forms of the BDEFS-CA.

CHAPTER 5

Relationship of BDEFS-CA Scores to Demographic Factors in the Normative Sample

This chapter describes the relationship of various demographic factors to the BDEFS-CA scores from both the long form and short form for the normative sample of 1,800 children.

Age

Age was correlated significantly with just three of the eight scores from the long form and one from the short form. Even then the correlations were of an exceptionally low magnitude, accounting for less than 5% of the variance. The significant correlations were (N = 1,800): Self-Management to Time (r = .07, p = .003); Self-Restraint (r = –.05, p = .045); Self-Regulation of Emotion (r = –.05, p = .026); EF Symptom Count for the Short Form (r = .06, p = .007).

However, correlation analyses may disguise nonlinear effects within such data. The relationships of age to the BDEFS-CA scores were therefore also analyzed using one-way analysis of variance (ANOVA) with the original 12 age groupings (6–17 years). The results were much the same. Significant effects of age were found on just one score, that being the EF Symptom Count for the Short Form of the BDEFS-CA: F = 1.84, p = .043. Even then, pairwise contrasts (Student Newman–Keuls) showed that this difference was significant (p < .05) only between the 7-year-olds (M = 1.9) and the 16-year-olds (M = 3.6), with no other pairwise age group comparisons being significant. One other score was marginally significant, that being the Self-Regulation of Emotion score: $F = 1.63$, $p = .085$. The results for each subscale score and the total score for the short form are shown in Figure 5.1. Here it is evident that there are no obvious (or significant) effects across the age groups. The pattern is essentially the same for the other scores from the long and short forms. This was not the case with the BRIEF rating scale for children, on which significant age effects were reported (Gioia et al., 2000). The differences in results may have to do with differences in item contents of the scales. The results here mean that, in presenting the norms, relatively large groupings of children can be made based on age ranges without obscuring any potentially significant age differences. The larger the age groupings that can be formed, the larger the sample sizes will be, and so the greater is the likelihood that the norms so presented are more reliable and representative of the U.S. population.

The findings at first glance may seem puzzling given the substantial effects of age found on many EF tests (see Chapter 1). However, it is highly likely that, when evaluating the EF items on the BDEFS-CA, parents are automatically adjusting for the age of the children in judging the child's EF difficulties; that is, they are judging their children against same-age peers. Although the instructions for completing the

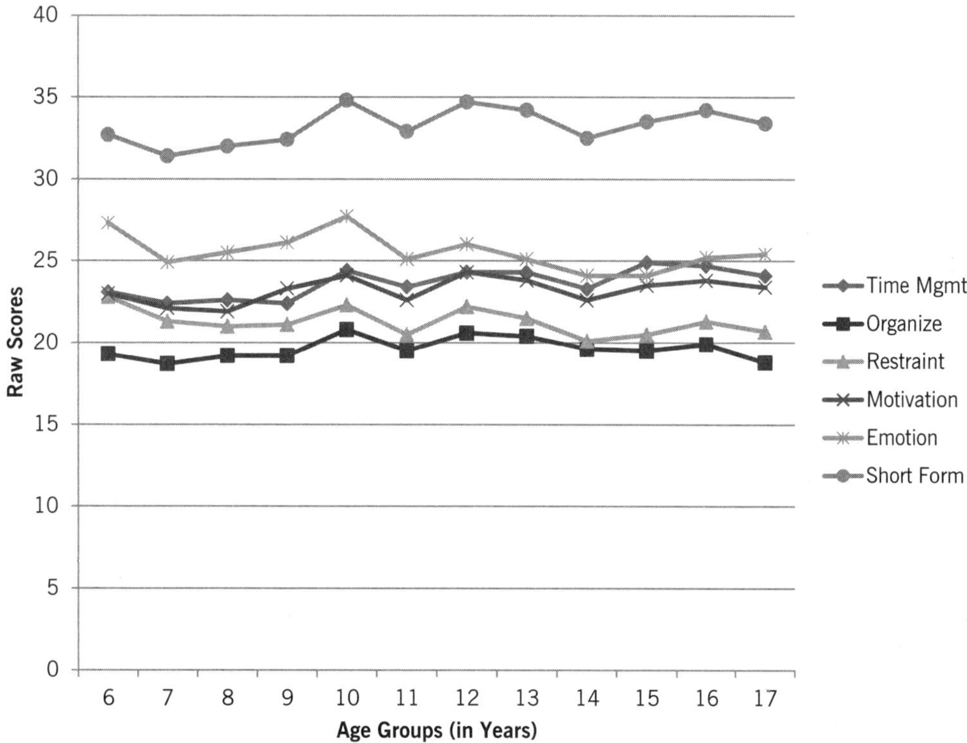

FIGURE 5.1. Raw scores for the 12 age groups for the five BDEFS-CA subscale scores from the long form and for the Total EF Summary Score for the short form. Time Mgmt, Self-Management to Time subscale; Organize, Self-Organization/Problem Solving subscale; Restraint, Self-Restraint subscale; Motivation, Self-Motivation subscale; Emotion, Self-Regulation of Emotion subscale.

scale do not tell parents to do so, 4 of the 70 items on the scale explicitly instruct parents to make such a comparison, for example, "Not as creative or inventive as others of his/her age." Therefore, the scores across the age levels may already be age-adjusted by the parents in making their judgments about how often their children demonstrate any particular EF problem (item). Of course, it is also possible that various EF difficulties or deficits are relatively stable across development, as is reflected in the relatively modest relationships between age and the EF scores as reported earlier. This might mean that children with EF difficulties retain their relative position in the population relative to other children of the same age across their development, although this cannot be directly evaluated in a cross-sectional study such as this one.

In view of these results showing a lack of significant age effects across the 12 narrow age levels, it was decided to cluster the age groups into two large age ranges of 6–11 ($N = 902$) and 12–17 ($N = 898$), representing childhood and adolescence, for the sake of presenting the norms and constructing the score sheets. This is similar to what was done with other scales assessing symptoms of child psychopathology, such as the Child Behavior Checklist (Achenbach, 2001), and for much the same reasons. When the analyses for age effects were repeated using the two large age groups instead of the 12 narrow age levels, the one-way ANOVAs indicated significant age differences for two scores from the long form: Self-Management to Time ($F = 7.86$, $p < .005$) and Self-Regulation of Emotion ($F = 5.26$, $p = .022$). There was also a significant age effect for the EF Symptom Count from the Short Form, $F = 5.38$, $p = .021$. The EF Summary Score for the short form was also marginally significant, $F = 3.48$, $p = .062$. These main effects are shown in Table 5.1. Such effects support the position taken here that norms should be presented employing these two large age groupings.

Sex Differences for Parents and Children

One-way ANOVAs were employed to compare the ratings of mothers and fathers ($N = 900$ each) on all 10 of the EF scores. None of the comparisons were significant. These results are similar to those reported for the BRIEF parent rating scale (Gioia et al., 2000), on which no significant effects in ratings were related to sex of the parent.

A comparison of the 901 males with the 899 females from the normative sample ($N = 1{,}800$) indicated significant sex differences on all of the scores except that for the Self-Regulation of Emotion subscale, which was marginally significant ($p = .094$). In each case, boys were rated as having slightly but significantly more problems than girls. The mean differences were small, as can be seen from Figure 5.2. This figure shows the raw scores for the five subscales of the BDEFS-CA Long Form and the EF Summary Score for the Short Form. The results for the other scores not portrayed in this graph were quite similar. Despite such small differences in means, their significance would indicate that at the extreme ends of the distributions different scores may have very different percentile ranks between the sexes that could be clinically meaningful. Sex differences between children were also found for the BRIEF rating scale of EF for children (Gioia et al., 2000), not to mention those

TABLE 5.1. BDEFS-CA Results for Each Sex within Each of the Two Age Groups Used to Create the EF Profiles in the Appendix

	Age groups × sex									
	6–11 years				12–17 years					
	Males		Females		Males		Females			
Subscale	Mean	*SD*	Mean	*SD*	Mean	*SD*	Mean	*SD*	*F*	*p*
Time Mgmt.	23.9	8.8	22.2	8.0	25.5	9.6	23.0	8.6	G = 7.93	.005
									S = 25.75	< .001
									G × S = 1.06	NS
Organization	19.9	7.6	19.0	7.0	20.5	8.5	19.1	7.0	G = 0.70	NS
									S = 10.75	.001
									G × S = 0.41	NS
Self-Restraint	22.7	8.8	20.4	7.9	21.7	9.0	20.4	8.0	G = 1.36	NS
									S = 21.48	< .001
									G × S = 1.47	NS
Self-Motivation	24.1	9.6	21.6	8.8	25.0	10.8	22.1	9.0	G = 2.47	NS
									S = 35.87	< .001
									G × S = 0.35	NS
Emotion Reg.	26.9	11.3	25.4	10.9	25.1	10.8	24.9	10.3	G = 5.27	.022
									S = 2.81	NS
									G × S = 1.51	NS
EF Summary Score	117.5	41.1	108.6	37.8	117.9	43.7	109.4	37.9	G = 0.08	NS
									S = 20.94	< .001
									G × S = 0.01	NS
ADHD EF Index	16.0	5.5	14.9	5.2	16.0	6.1	14.8	5.1	G = 0.02	NS
									S = 18.32	< .001
									G × S=0.10	NS
EF Symptom Count	10.0	15.8	7.4	13.5	10.9	16.7	7.7	13.4	G = 0.75	NS
									S = 17.18	< .001
									G × S = 0.15	NS
Short Form—EF Summary Score	33.9	11.7	31.5	10.9	35.0	12.7	32.5	11.2	G = 3.50	.062
									S = 19.64	< .001
									G × S = 0.03	NS
Short Form—EF Symptom Count	2.9	4.6	2.2	4.0	3.6	5.0	2.6	4.1	G = 5.40	.020
									S = 16.53	< .001
									G × S = 0.59	NS

Note. Time Mgmt., Self-Management to Time subscale; Organization, Self-Organization/Problem Solving subscale; Emotion Reg., Self-Regulation of Emotion subscale; EF Summary, Total EF Summary score; *F*, results for the *F*-test from the ANOVA; G, main effect for age group; S, main effect for sex; G × S, interaction of age group × sex; *p*, probability value for each of the *F*-tests if ≤ .05; NS, not significant.

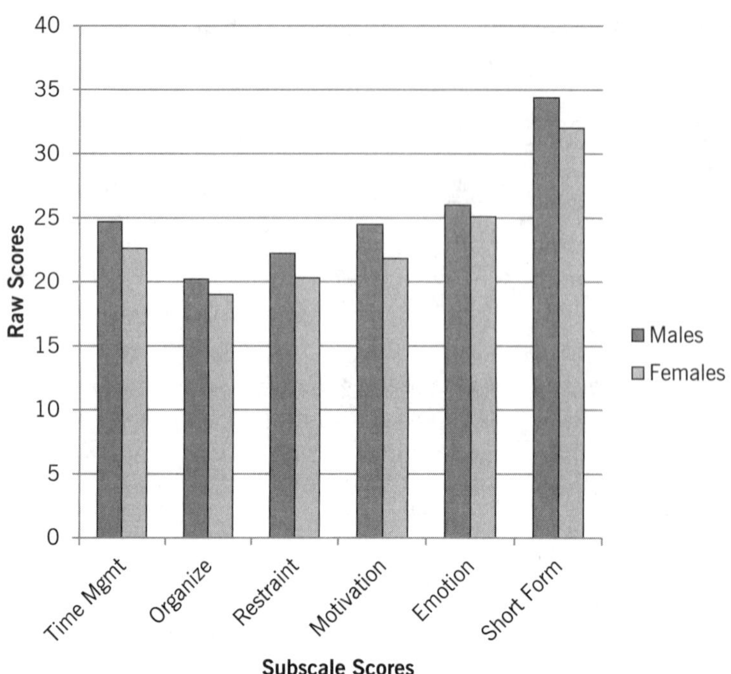

FIGURE 5.2. Raw scores for the five BDEFS-CA subscale raw scores from the long form and the short form total raw score. Time Mgmt = Self-Management to Time subscale; Organize, Self-Organization/Problem-Solving subscale; Restraint, Self-Restraint subscale; Motivation, Self-Motivation subscale; Emotion, Self-Regulation of Emotion subscale.

scales assessing symptoms of child psychopathology (Achenbach, 2001; Reynolds & Kamphaus, 2004). Therefore, norms are presented separately for each sex on the EF Profiles provided in the Appendix.

Using the normative sample, the next analyses examined whether there was an interaction of age with sex on any of the BDEFS-CA scales. Two-way analyses of variance (sex × 12 age groups) were applied to each of the 10 scores from the BDEFS-CA scales. In no instance was there any significant interaction of age group with sex. These analyses were repeated using the 2 large age groups rather than the 12 narrow ones. The results were the same in that there was no significant age-by-sex interaction. The results of those analyses are shown in Table 5.1. Consequently, the norms are presented on the score sheets for the two sexes within the two large age groupings of 6–11 and 12–17 years. This resulted in norms being available for 451 males and 451 females between 6 and 11 years of age and 450 males and 448 females between 12 and 17 years of age.

Ethnic Group

The next issue to address in considering how to best portray the norms for scoring purposes concerned whether there exists any significant relationship of ethnic group to the BDEFS-CA scores. One-way ANOVAs revealed no significant effects of ethnic group on any of the scores, nor did any comparisons even approach marginal significance ($p < .10$). This has also been the case with other EF rating scales for use with parents (Gioia et al., 2000). Consequently, there seems to be little or no clinical value to scoring the BDEFS-CA in displaying the norms for each ethnic group. All ethnic groups were therefore collapsed together in the portrayal of the norms on the EF Profiles in the Appendix.

Parent Education and Household Income

Correlations were computed between the educational levels of the respondent parents in the normative sample and all 10 of the EF scores. Low but significant relationships were found for the following eight scores: Self-Management to Time ($r = -.05$, $p = .032$); Self-Organization/Problem Solving ($r = -.10$, $p < .001$); Self-Motivation ($r = -.07$, $p = .004$); EF Summary Score ($r = -.06$, $p = .007$); ADHD EF Index ($r = -.07$, $p = .004$); EF Symptom Count ($r = -.09$, $p < .001$); Short Form EF Summary Score ($r = -.07$, $p = .004$); and Short Form EF Symptom Count ($r = -.10$, $p < .001$). The correlations for the Self-Restraint and Self-Regulation of Emotion scores were not significant. In each instance parents with less education reported somewhat higher EF deficits in their children. The relationships are quite small, though significant, and indicate that the shared variance between parent education and the EF scores is 1% or less. The correlations between the educational levels of the nonrespondent parents and these same 10 scores were similar, though slightly higher in magnitude, and ranged from –.04 (not significant) to –.14 (Self-Organization, $p < .001$). The same results were evident for the correlations between household income level and the EF scores. In this case, all but one of the correlations reached significance. The correlations ranged from only –.06 to –.10. Again, the shared variance here is less than 1% and of little consequence for the reporting of the normative results. The same low but significant relationships between EF scores and parent education and income have been reported for other parent rating scales of EF (Gioia et al., 2000). These relationships are likely significant owing to the large sample size used here ($N = 1{,}800$). If anything, such findings may provide modest evidence of validity in that greater difficulties with EF in children, just as with symptoms of child psychopathology, would be expected to be somewhat greater in the lowest educational and income groups. As a result, the educational and income levels were collapsed together for portrayal of the norms.

Geographic Region

Potential differences in the scores from the scale with regard to geographic regions were evaluated using one-way ANOVA comparing the four major regions of the United States using the normative sample (N=1,800). There were no significant differences for any of the scores for either the long form or the short form, nor did any of the scores even approach marginal significance. It is therefore reasonable to collapse the geographic regions together for purposes of displaying the normative information on this sample.

Conclusion

In view of the preceding findings and discussion, separate EF Profiles are provided in the Appendix that contain the various raw scores from the long form and their associated percentiles for males ages 6–11 (N = 451), males ages 12–17 (N = 450), females ages 6–11 (N = 451), and females ages 12–17 (N = 448). Additional EF Profiles show the separate norms for each of these groups for the two scores that can be computed from the short form.

CHAPTER 6

Reliability

This brief chapter presents the information that is available concerning the various forms of reliability regarding the BDEFS-CA. Obviously, more research on these and other psychometric characteristics of the scale is to be encouraged. But what information is available indicates that the reliabilities of the scale scores are satisfactory and support the use of the BDEFS-CA in clinical practice and research where the assessment of parental reports concerning EF deficits in daily life activities in their children is of interest.

Subscale Relationships

As indicated by the factor analysis reported earlier, ratings of EF in daily life activities appear to tap a large underlying dimension that mainly represents self-regulation. That dimension can be further broken down into five interrelated components or types of self-regulation (Self-Organization, Self-Management to Time, Self-Restraint, Self-Motivation, and Self-Regulation of Emotion). We should therefore not be surprised to find that the BDEFS-CA scales created from these dimensions are likewise interrelated yet partially separable. In one sense, this quality reflects a form of internal consistency of the scale. Are the subscales sufficiently related to each other so as to be clustered under the metaconstruct of EF?

The relationships among the scales were evaluated using Pearson product–moment correlations on the entire original sample of 1,922 participants. The results are shown in Table 6.1 and indicate that the scales were significantly ($p < .001$) and moderately to highly intercorrelated. The strongest relationships were between the Self-Restraint and Self-Regulation of Emotion subscales (.83) and between the

TABLE 6.1. Intercorrelations among the BDEFS-CA Long Form Subscales

Scales	1	2	3	4	5	6
1. Time Mgmt.	1.00					
2. Organization	.69	1.00				
3. Self-Restraint	.76	.69	1.00			
4. Motivation	.84	.70	.81	1.00		
5. Emotion Reg.	.64	.63	.83	.75	1.00	
6. ADHD Index	.82	.86	.88	.89	.84	1.00

Note. Time Mgmt., Self-Management to Time subscale; Organization, Self-Organization/Problem Solving subscale; Motivation, Self-Motivation subscale; Emotion Reg., Self-Regulation of Emotion subscale. Analyses: Pearson product–moment correlations. All correlations are statistically significant at $p < .001$.

Self-Management to Time and Self-Motivation subscales (.84). The former relationship is understandable given that the initial step in emotional self-control has been argued to be inhibition, followed by subsequent efforts at self-management of the emotional state, as discussed in earlier chapters (Gross, 1998). The weakest relationships occurred between the Self-Management to Time and the Self-Regulation of Emotion subscales (.64) and between the Self-Organization/Problem Solving and Self-Regulation of Emotion subscales (.63). The shared variance among the scales ranges from 39 to 70%. This implies that there is likely an underlying unitary construct of EF, as found in the PCFA in Chapter 4, perhaps comparable to *g* in research on intelligence tests. Yet some unique variance is accounted for by each scale apart from the others. The ADHD-EF Index score also correlated highly with each of the five subscale scores from the BDEFS-CA Long Form, which is not surprising given that one or more of its items are drawn from each of these subscales. The BDEFS-CA Short Form EF Summary Score was found to correlate highly with the same score from the full BDEFS-CA Long Form: $r = .98$ ($p < .001$); indicating that the short form score is a very good approximation of the results that would be obtained from the longer version of the scale. This was also the case for the EF Symptom Count score from both forms: $r = .97$ ($p < .001$).

Internal Consistency

The internal consistency (Cronbach's alpha) of each BDEFS-CA Long Form subscale was computed based on the entire sample of 1,922 and found to be quite satisfactory: Self-Management to Time ($r = .956$), Self-Organization/Problem Solving ($r = .956$), Self-Restraint ($r = .955$), Self-Motivation ($r = .965$), and Self-Regulation of Emotion ($r = .972$). For the ADHD-EF Index, it was $r = .904$. For the entire 70-item long form, it was $r = .987$. For the short form 20-item scale, it was $r = .953$. All *F*-tests were significant at $p < .001$. Such results are quite comparable to other rating scales of EF in children (Gioia et al., 2000) and to the adult version of the BDEFS (Barkley, 2011a). Thus the internal consistency of the subscales is quite satisfactory.

Test–Retest Reliability

Test–retest reliability reflects the temporal consistency of a measure. It was assessed by having a subset of the original sample complete the scale on a second occasion 3–5 weeks after initially completing the scale. A total of 86 parents completed the scale a second time, with at least 5 children for each age level from 6–17 years. There were 45 boys and 41 girls in this sample. The breakdown for the sex of the parent was 36 males and 50 females. These parents were randomly chosen by Knowledge Networks within each age group and sex and invited to return to the website to complete the scale for a second time. They were, of course, paid for their participation, just as were all participants on the first occasion of assessment.

The Pearson product–moment correlations between the first and second administrations were: Self-Management to Time, .73 ($p < .001$); Self-Organization/Problem Solving, .77 ($p < .001$); Self-Restraint, .77 ($p < .001$); Self-Motivation, .78 ($p < .001$); Self-Regulation of Emotion, .82 ($p < .001$); and the Total EF Summary Score, .82 ($p < .001$). The test–retest reliability for the ADHD-EF Index was .79 ($p < .001$); and for the BDEFS-CA Short Form EF Summary Score was .79 ($p < .001$). These results are quite satisfactory and indicate a reasonable level of test–retest reliability over this 3- to 5-week period. They are also relatively comparable to the test–retest reliability found for other rating scales of EF for children, such as the BRIEF, which used a 2-week retest period and found an average reliability of 0.81 (range .76–.85) (Gioia et al., 2000). Research has also found the test–retest reliability of the CHEXI rating scale to be .89 over a 2-week interval (Thorell & Nyberg, 2008).

The actual scores from the initial testing and retesting administrations were then compared using a paired-samples *t*-test. The results are shown in Table 6.2. They indicate that the subscale scores, EF Summary Score, and ADHD-EF Index score from the long form and the EF Summary Score from the short form did not

TABLE 6.2. Comparison of Initial and Retesting Sample Results on the BDEFS-CA Long and Short Form Scores ($N = 86$)

	Initial		Retesting		Mean		
Subscale	Mean	SD	Mean	SD	diff.	*t*	*p*
Self-Management to Time	23.1	8.3	23.6	9.0	+0.4	0.64	NS
Self-Organization	18.7	6.7	19.8	8.1	+1.1	1.97	NS
Self-Restraint	21.0	8.9	21.2	9.0	+0.2	0.36	NS
Self-Motivation	23.4	9.6	23.2	10.7	−0.2	0.28	NS
Self-Reg. of Emotion	25.6	11.5	25.7	11.2	+0.1	0.05	NS
Total EF Summary Score	111.9	40.6	113.5	43.9	+1.6	0.58	NS
ADHD-EF Index	15.3	5.6	15.4	6.0	+0.1	0.32	NS
EF Summary Score Short Form	32.7	11.9	33.2	12.6	+0.5	0.52	NS

Note. Mean diff., differences in the initial and retesting means; *t*, results for the paired-samples *t*-test; *p*, probability value for the *t*-test if ≤.05; NS, not significant; Self-Organization, Self-Organization/Problem Solving subscale; Self-Reg. of Emotion, Self-Regulation of Emotion subscale.

change significantly across this 3- to 5-week test–retest interval. The change in the Self-Organization/Problem Solving subscale score was marginally significant, however ($p = .052$). Again, this supports the conclusion that both the BDEFS-CA Long and Short Forms have satisfactory test–retest reliability (stability) with no evidence of significant changes in scale results over this interval of time.

Conclusion

The BDEFS-CA has quite satisfactory levels of various forms of internal, as well as cross-temporal, consistency (test–retest reliability). The findings are sufficient to support the use of the BDEFS-CA as a reliable measure of EF in the daily life activities of children.

CHAPTER 7

Validity

This chapter presents the information that is available concerning several important forms of validity for the scores from the BDEFS-CA. Information on the relationship of the scale to impairment measures is presented in Chapter 8. As with the information on reliability in the previous chapter, more research on these forms of validity and other psychometric characteristics of the scale is to be welcomed. Nevertheless, the current information available and discussed herein indicates that the validity of the scale is quite reasonable and acceptable. Such information supports the use of the BDEFS-CA in clinical practice and research when the assessment of parental reports concerning EF deficits in daily life activities in their children is of interest.

The term "validity" typically refers to the correctness, accuracy, or truth of an assertion or conclusion as judged against the empirical evidence (Bryant, 2000). In this instance of measurement development, it refers to the extent to which the rating scale measures what it claims to assess. To what extent is the BDEFS-CA measuring EF in the daily life activities of children? And to what degree is it useful in doing so? Much of the work of validating the BDEFS-CA was done over the previous decade with the prototype version of the adult scale and with the subsequent final form (Barkley, 2011a). The content of the adult and parent scales is highly similar in that nearly all of the items on each of the subscales of the BDEFS-CA were derived from the comparable subscale of the adult form. As reviewed in the manual for the BDEFS adult scale (Barkley, 2011a), the evidence for the reliability and validity of the adult scale is substantial. Ratings on the adult scale are significantly associated with impairment in numerous domains of adult functioning in which EF should be operative, such as education, work, driving, marriage, criminal behavior, drug use, health concerns, parenting stress, offspring psychological maladjustment, and general ratings of overall impairment, among others. Various groups formed on the basis of these and other risk factors, as well as of adult psychiatric disorders, such as adult ADHD, differed significantly in their BDEFS scores. Given that the BDEFS-CA contains highly similar items to the adult scale, with some rephrasing for application to children, there is every reason to believe that the child and adolescent form of the BDEFS would be found to have substantial validity as well. What evidence is available is fairly substantial and is discussed herein. It is satisfactory and supports the use of this scale as a measure of EF deficits in daily life activities in children ages 6–17 years.

Construct Validity

As noted by others, construct validity starts with an explicit definition of the construct that a measure is intended to assess (Bryant, 2000; Cook & Campbell, 1979). Otherwise, one cannot determine whether the measure is accurately or correctly sampling from and hence evaluating the conceptual (semantic) domain of this construct. This form of validity may also be known as conceptual or content validity. Despite the widespread use of the term "executive functioning" or "EF," it has not been especially well defined and lacks a consensus definition, as noted earlier (Chapter 1) and elsewhere (Barkley, 2012b). Therefore any effort to evaluate the construct validity of any measure of EF has been hampered by the ambiguity in and lack of any agreement about the definition of the term. However, unlike other rating scales of EF, the items on the BDEFS adult and child forms were developed from a theory of EF (Barkley, 1997a). That theory views EF as comprising acts of self-regulation that are used to modify one's own behavior so as to alter the likelihood of delayed or later outcomes—it is future-directed action (Barkley, 1997a, 1997c, 2012b). Its components consist of various forms of self-directed actions that humans use to choose goals and to select, enact, and sustain behavior across time toward those goals, typically in the context of others and often using social and cultural means (Barkley, 2012a). Based on this definition of EF, the BDEFS-CA has high conceptual or face validity in that its items were chosen to reflect the major components of this theory of EF: (1) inhibition (self-restraint); (2) nonverbal working memory (largely visual–spatial imagery) and its use in hindsight, foresight, sense of time, and self-management to time; (3) verbal working memory (self-directed speech) and its use in planning, problem solving, and rule-governed (symbolically guided) behavior; (4) self-regulation of emotion and motivation; and (5) reconstitution or goal-directed innovation and creativity. Items for the scale were also based on a review of the relevant literature pertaining to the deficits believed to be associated with the dysexecutive syndrome and the most frequently identified constructs believed to be subsumed under the rubric of EF (see Chapter 1).

A form of validity related to construct validity is convergent validity. Do various measures of the same construct converge or agree? Most other measures of EF are tests or psychometric instruments. Indeed, it would appear from the frequency with which they are used in research and clinical practice that they are the sole or gold standard for evaluating the EF construct and its components. Should they be so esteemed?

Relationship to EF Tests

As a consequence of their numerous inherent problems, discussed in Chapter 1 and elsewhere (Barkley, 2011a, 2012b), it is obvious that EF tests cannot be used as the sole or gold standard against which to evaluate a new measure of EF, in this case a rating scale of EF in children's everyday life activities. It is questionable whether the wide array of tests claimed to be evaluating EF in neuropsychology meet acceptable standards themselves for construct validity, much less serve as the standard against which any new measure of EF is to be judged. As previously noted, tests of EF are poorly correlated with rating scales of EF (see Chapter 1) and are equally poor at predicting functioning and impairment in major life activities in which EF would be considered to be indispensable. As I argued previously (Barkley, 2011a), EF tests should not be the standard for evaluating the construct validity of a new measure of EF, especially a rating scale, given the substantial evidence already available as to their own low construct, and especially ecological, validity. The prevailing evidence suggests that the problem rests with the tests more than with the rating scales of EF, especially if predicting functioning and impairment in major life activities is the clinical objective in the evaluation of EF.

As noted previously, past research with the adult version of the BDEFS did examine its relationship to several different batteries of EF tests (Barkley & Fischer, 2011; Barkley & Murphy, 2011). The results found that subscales were modestly but significantly related to some EF tests but not significantly related to others. The BDEFS scales shared less than 10% of their variance with such tests at best and less than 20% with any best combination of EF tests (for analyses, see Barkley, 2011a; Barkley & Fischer, 2011; Barkley & Murphy, 2011). This cannot be blamed on the relatively small test batteries or on the particular choice of EF tests. The results were very consistent with a number of other previous studies that used other EF tests and rating scales and found much the same results (see Chapter 2; see also McAuley, Chen, Goos, Schachar, & Crosbie, 2010; Roth, Isquith, & Gioia, 2005; Zandt et al., 2009). Hence the limited relationship of EF ratings to EF tests poses more of a problem for the construct and ecological validity of the tests than it shows evidence of a problem with EF rating scales such as the BDEFS-CA. Some have mistakenly drawn the opposite conclusion from the limited relationship between EF ratings and EF tests (McAuley et al., 2010). But the proof of validity here lies in the prediction of impairment in major life activities in which EF is presumed to be essential; and on that count, EF ratings far surpass EF tests.

No research is yet available on the relationships of the BDEFS-CA to various neuropsychological tests presumed to evaluate EF. Nevertheless, those relationships would be expected to be of a low magnitude, just as has been found for the adult version of the BDEFS, noted previously. This would also be inferred from research on other rating scales of EF deficits in children that evaluated their relationship to psychometric EF tests (Anderson et al., 2002; Goulden & Silver, 2009; Mahone et al., 2002; McAuley et al., 2010; Thorell & Nyberg, 2008; Zandt et al., 2009). In those studies, correlations ranged from just .01 to .48, were often not significant, and usually fell in the .20–.30 range, sharing less than 10% of their variance on average. EF ratings and EF tests are clearly not measuring the same construct. EF ratings are also more strongly related to measures of adaptive functioning, psychopathology, and educational performance and school adjustment, as well as other domains of impairment, than are EF tests (Barkley & Fischer, 2011; Barkley & Murphy, 2010; Mahone et al., 2002; see also Chapter 1).

Relationship to Other EF Rating Scales

In contrast to EF tests, other rating scales of EF can be used as a more direct indication of the construct (convergent) validity of the BDEFS-CA. The only other commercially available rating scale of EF deficits for children that has a large normative sample is the BRIEF (Gioia et al., 2000). For this manual, the BRIEF and BDEFS-CA were completed by the same parents for 22 children, ages 6–17 years, with approximately equal representation of males and females. This was a sample of convenience from parents in the southern and northeastern United States. It included children with psychiatric and learning disorders, as well as children without disorders, thus ensuring an adequate range of scores on the measures. The three factor-based scores from the BRIEF (Behavior Regulation, Metacognition, and Total EF Score) were correlated with the five factor-based subscale scores and EF Summary Score from the BDEFS-CA Long Form. The results are shown in Table 7.1. The correlations are significant and of a moderate to high magnitude. Indeed, the relationship between the EF total scores from both scales is of such a high magnitude (r = .92) as to indicate virtual colinearity (both scales are measuring precisely the same domain). Also noteworthy is the fact that the Behavior Regulation domain of the BRIEF is most highly related to the Self-Restraint and Self-Regulation of Emotion domains on the BDEFS-CA. This ought to be the case given that the Behavior Regulation Index is composed of symptoms of both inhibition and emotion regulation. The Metacognitive Index score of the BRIEF is most highly related to the Self-Management to Time and Self-Motivation subscales of the BDEFS-CA, demonstrat-

TABLE 7.1. Correlations of BDEFS-CA Scores with Factor-Based Scores from the BRIEF for 22 Children

	BRIEF scales[b]		
BDEFS-CA scales[a]	Beh. Reg.	Metacognition	Total EF Score
Time Management	.58	.90	.86
Self-Organization	.60	.53	.59
Self-Restraint	.80	.69	.78
Self-Motivation	.63	.77	.79
Emotion Self-Reg.	.78	.64	.74
EF Summary Score	.83	.87	.92

Note. Analyses: Pearson product–moment correlations. All correlations are statistically significant at $p < .001$.
[a]Time Management = Self-Management to Time subscale; Self-Organization, Self-Organization/Problem Solving subscale; Emotion Self-Reg., Self-Regulation of Emotion subscale.
[b]Beh. Reg., Behavioral Regulation Scale; Metacognition, Metacognitive Index Scale.

ing significant conceptual overlap among these dimensions and again consistent with expectations given the overlapping item contents of these respective scales. These results also imply that the substantial research that exists on the validity of the BRIEF for children could be extrapolated to the BDEFS-CA as well.

Evidence from Factor Analyses

Some evidence of how well the BDEFS-CA captures EF became evident in the research conducted over the past decade with the adult; BDEFS and its factor or dimensional content (Barkley, 2011a; Barkley et al., 2008; Barkley & Fischer, 2011; Barkley & Murphy, 2010, 2011). This research provides an indication as well of the content or conceptual validity of the scale. Do its items form dimensions that are believed to be major forms of EF in daily life, as described in the theory used to create the items? A factor analysis of the initial prototype of the adult BDEFS using a mixed sample of ADHD, clinical, and community control groups identified factors that are highly consistent with the initial theory of EF used to create the scale, as well as with descriptions of the deficits often associated with various forms of PFC injury or maldevelopment. These dimensions were initially labeled as Self-Management to Time, Self-Organization/Problem Solving, Self-Inhibition (Self-Discipline), Self-Motivation, and Self-Activation. This same factor structure emerged from the ratings of others on the same scale concerning the adult participants in that study (Barkley & Murphy, 2011). And it emerged again in a longitudinal study of hyperactive children concerning the persistence of their ADHD into young adulthood (Barkley & Fischer, 2011) that employed an interview version of the BDEFS. The final version of the BDEFS was normed using a substantial sample of adults who were representative of the U.S. population (more than 1,200) and likewise found four of these five same factors, with the exception of the Self-Activation factor. That factor was considerably weaker and comprised just a few items. Hence it was omitted from further consideration in development of the final version of the BDEFS for adults. It likely emerged in the earlier studies related to ADHD because such problems with self-activation may be particularly problematic for that clinical disorder whereas they are not so evident in a general population sample. The four factors were also identified in the study by Fedele and colleagues (2010) using a substantial sample of college students. It therefore appears that the factor structure of the BDEFS with regard to dimensions representing Self-Management to Time, Self-Organization/Problem Solving, Self-Restraint, and Self-Motivation are reliable features of EF in daily life.

No factor related to emotional self-regulation had the opportunity to emerge in the past research using the prototype of the adult BDEFS as items assessing that aspect of EF were not included in that prototype—an oversight that was corrected in the subsequent and final version of the BDEFS (Barkley, 2011a) and in the present parent-report version. That correction proved fruitful, as the subsequent factor analysis of the adult normative sample (Barkley, 2011a) and the present child and adolescent sample both revealed just such a dimension of EF in daily life activities. It was a factor comprising items dealing with problems with emotional inhibition and self-regulation, just as would be expected from Gross's modal model of emotional self-regulation (see Chapter 2).

All of these efforts to identify the underlying dimensions of the initial large item pool of EF symptoms in daily life suggest that the BDEFS-CA has reasonable construct, conceptual, or content validity, as well as convergent validity, when judged against the definition of EF offered in Chapter 1 and against other rating scales of EF deficits. The BDEFS-CA does appear to be assessing self-regulation across time to attain future goals, at least as that may be reflected in survey items focusing on specific forms of behavior involved in such self-regulation. The BDEFS-CA is a theoretically, not just an empirically, based rating scale of EF developed specifically from a particular conceptualization of EF.

It will also prove informative for research to evaluate the extent to which various groups having psychiatric and neurological disorders perform on the BDEFS-CA. Some research with children so diagnosed in this normative sample will be noted shortly. But it is not essential for the construct validity of the BDEFS-CA to be shown to discriminate patients with frontal lobe disorders as a sine qua non for its construct validity unless one wishes to regress to an earlier era of research on EF when it was chiefly believed to represent "what the frontal lobes do." As Denckla (1996) has previously noted, conflating EF with any neurological substrate confuses levels of analysis in science (psychological with the neurological) and does not provide a solid conceptual basis on which to further develop and evaluate the concept of EF at the neuropsychological level of analysis.

Divergent or Discriminant Validity

We turn now to evidence of divergent or discriminant validity. As Bryant (2000) has explained, this refers to evidence that the construct of EF as evaluated by the BDEFS-CA differs from other psychological constructs that it is not intended to evaluate or measure. It is the opposite of convergent validity, in which measures of the same construct ought to converge on or correlate with one another, as discussed earlier.

Relationship to IQ

EF is not considered to be an identical construct to intelligence, or IQ. Given how they are conceptualized, one might expect a modest relationship between them in that some aspects of EF, such as working memory, may be contained within some IQ tests. But the field of neuropsychology generally treats these as distinct concepts. It is therefore important to show that the BDEFS is largely not contaminated with intelligence. No evidence currently exists on the relationship of the parent-report form of the BDEFS-CA with measures of IQ. But prior findings with the adult form of the BDEFS found that it was not significantly associated with IQ to any appreciable degree across ages 18–81 years (Barkley, 2011a; Barkley & Murphy, 2011). The range of correlations between the various BDEFS scores and IQ was shown to be just –.04 to –.17, with most not being statistically significant. Essentially, adult ratings of EF shared less than 2% of their variance with measures of IQ. The same would be expected for the parent-report form. This issue, as noted previously, has posed a considerable problem for EF tests. They are often contaminated by their significant overlap with general intelligence or with other cognitive constructs not believed to represent EF, such as motor, processing, or naming speed.

Relationship to Academic Achievement Tests

EF is also conceptualized as a distinctly different construct from academic achievement, which essentially reflects the level of knowledge of particular academic subjects someone possesses. This is not to say that EF is unimportant to the acquisition of academic knowledge, only that it is not intended to represent that end state of acquired information. Past research with the adult BDEFS found it to be correlated modestly with academic achievement skills, as measured by the Wide Range Achievement Test (WRAT; Jastak & Wilkinson, 1993), as one might expect. But the relationships are low and often nonsignificant (range .12–.16). Yet even where the relationships were significant, they were weak and indicated that the BDEFS scales shared less than 3% of their variance with certain achievement skills. No research has yet been done on the relationship of the BDEFS-CA to academic achievement tests in children. Past research on other child rating scales of EF deficits, such as the CHEXI, found a range of correlations of –.11 to –.42 for mathematics and –.16 to –.46 for language skills (Thorell & Nyberg, 2008). Most of these relationships were significant as might be expected given the importance of EF components such as working memory and resistance to distraction to performance on such academic tests and to knowledge acquisition. Yet even here the overlap in variance is less than 21%, clearly indicating that EF and achievement are not identical constructs. Much the same would be expected from the BDEFS-CA given its substantial content overlap with other child EF rating scales such as the BRIEF, with which it is highly correlated if not collinear (see earlier discussion).

Criterion Validity: Differentiating among Disorders

Another form of validity that is important to the clinical utility of a measure is the extent to which the measure predicts a well-accepted indicator of that construct. As Bryant (2000) explained, if a measure is valid at assessing a construct such as EF, then it should be shown to be related to past, present, and future measures or outcomes believed to be associated with that construct.

Such evidence can come from studies of a scale's capacity to distinguish among disordered and normal groups when those disordered groups are believed to vary in the extent to which they have problems with EF. EF is such a highly important and ubiquitously employed human adaptation, as one of a human's principal means of survival (Barkley, 2012b), that it is likely to be disrupted by a variety of human ailments or disorders. Yet the impact of such adverse conditions would be expected to vary in degree and, given the multidimensional nature of EF, in patterning as well. As is discussed later, evidence suggests that most forms of developmental, learning, and psychiatric disorders interfere with one or more components of EF. But they are not hypothesized to do so to the same degree and with the same pattern of effects across EF dimensions. A valid measure of EF in daily life activities and its components should therefore demonstrate differential patterning across various disorders, reflecting the extent to which EF or any EF component is thought to be adversely affected by that disorder.

What follows is evidence for the criterion validity of the BDEFS-CA based on multiple developmental, learning, and psychiatric disorders present in the general population sample reported here. The findings also reveal new knowledge about the differential impact of various disorders on parent ratings of EF in the daily lives of children, which is important given that no prior studies have done so for many of these disorders. Even in the few disorders for which such evidence may be available, only one or a few studies exist, and thus the following evidence can serve as replication of those findings. Moreover, given that the structure of the BDEFS-CA is somewhat different from those of other EF rating scales, findings for the BDEFS-CA can serve to further extend that knowledge of EF deficits in daily life associated with those childhood disorders.

Neurodevelopmental Disorders

Attention-Deficit/Hyperactivity Disorder

ADHD is not just a childhood psychiatric disorder. It has been hypothesized to represent a developmental disorder of EF (Barkley, 1997a, 1997c) and to interfere with all of the components of EF, though not to the same degree across dimensions. The disorder has a large neurological contribution to its etiology and is understood to arise from either maldevelopment of or injury to the PFC and its networks (Barkley, 2006; Bush et al., 2005; Hutchinson et al., 2008; Mackie et al., 2007; Nigg, 2006; Paloyelis et al., 2007; Valera et al., 2007). Given that the PFC is the "executive brain," then it makes perfect logical sense that ADHD must be a disorder of EF. Evidence certainly shows that ADHD is associated with numerous difficulties in EF typically assessed using EF tests (Frazier et al., 2004; Hervey et al., 2004; Willcutt et al., 2005). Prior research with the adult BDEFS found that adults with ADHD have significantly higher ratings on all subscales of this scale than do community samples of adults (Barkley, 2011a; Barkley & Fischer, 2011; Barkley & Murphy, 2011). They also have higher ratings on the prototype of the BDEFS than do clinic-referred adults using self-report forms and other-reports of EF (Barkley & Murphy, 2011). And higher scores on the prototype of the BDEFS scales were associated with the degree of persistence of ADHD into adulthood in hyperactive children followed longitudinally in the Milwaukee Study, particularly relative to a Community control group (Barkley & Fischer, 2011). Consistent with theory, the vast majority of adults with ADHD (86–98%) were impaired (falling above the 93rd percentile) across the five dimensions of the BDEFS. Significant deficits in EF ratings in daily life activities have also been reported for adults and children with ADHD on other EF rating scales (Gioia et al., 2000; Joyner, Silver, & Stavinoha, 2009; Mahone & Hoffman, 2007; Roth et al., 2005). As indicated in Chapter 4, information was collected on the entire sample reported here for the BDEFS-CA with regard to past professional diagnoses of various developmental, learning, and psychiatric disorders. This information can be used to directly examine this type of criterion validity of the BDEFS-CA.

As noted in Chapter 4, ratings were collected on the extent of ADHD (DSM-IV) symptoms present in all participants in the original sample of 1,922 children. These ratings were correlated with the BDEFS-CA subscales or dimensions. The results are shown in Table 7.2. They indicated moderate to high relationships between ADHD inattention, ADHD hyperactive–impulsive, and total ADHD symptoms and all scales and summary scores from the BDEFS-CA, ranging from .70 to .88. Such findings support prior studies finding significant EF deficits associated with ADHD, especially when ratings of EF are employed (Barkley & Murphy, 2011; Reddy et al., 2011). The shared variance between ADHD symptoms and EF ratings is as high as 77% in this sample of children, as well as in the adult normative sample for the BDEFS (Barkley, 2011a). Those results support the prior conclusion that ADHD may well represent a disorder of EF rather than just one of inattention (Barkley, 1997a, 1997c; Barkley & Murphy, 2011).

An alternative means of demonstrating this relationship is to compare those children who had received a professional diagnosis of ADHD or ADD as reported by parents ($N = 173$) in the entire sample here with those who had not received such a diagnosis ($N = 1{,}749$). These comparisons are shown in Table 7.3. Significant and substantial differences were evident on all BDEFS-CA scores. As noted in Chapter 4, such reports of professional diagnoses are a less rigorous means of determining the presence of a psychiatric disorder than an approach in which the actual symptoms of the disorder and presence of impairment are determined directly with the parent, in this case by using actual DSM-IV symptoms. As just discussed, those symptoms and reports of impairment were collected from these parents. Taking this approach to the present sample, children were classified as having ADHD if they placed at the 93rd percentile or higher on either or both ADHD symptom lists

TABLE 7.2. Correlations of BDEFS-CA Scores with ADHD Ratings in the Total Sample (*N* = 1,922)

	ADHD scales		
BDEFS-CA scales	Inattention	Hyperactive–Impulsive	Total ADHD
Time Management	.80	.60	.76
Self-Organization	.74	.62	.74
Self-Restraint	.77	.73	.81
Self-Motivation	.88	.66	.83
Emotion Self-Reg.	.70	.67	.74
EF Summary Score	.87	.74	.87
ADHD EF Index	.87	.74	.87
EF Symptom Count	.82	.70	.82
EF Summary Score—Short Form	.86	.72	.85
EF Symptom Count—Short Form	.81	.68	.80

Note. Analyses: Pearson product–moment correlations. All correlations are statistically significant at $p < .001$. Time Management, Self-Management to Time subscale; Self-Organization, Self-Organization/Problem Solving subscale; Emotion Self-Reg., Self-Regulation of Emotion subscale.

TABLE 7.3. BDEFS-CA Long and Short Form Scores for Children in the Entire Sample Whose Parents Reported Having a Professional Diagnosis of ADHD/ADD and the Sample Remainder

	No ADHD/ADD (N= 1,749)		ADHD/ADD (N= 173)			
Subscale	Mean	*SD*	Mean	*SD*	*F*	*p*
Self-Management to Time	22.6	8.0	34.3	9.7	328.55	< .001
Self-Organization	18.8	6.6	27.6	10.7	240.17	< .001
Self-Restraint	20.2	7.4	31.8	10.7	351.22	< .001
Self-Motivation	22.0	8.5	35.4	11.2	363.90	< .001
Self-Reg. of Emotion	24.5	9.8	37.0	13.8	237.02	< .001
Total EF Summary Score	108.1	35.3	166.1	47.9	396.32	< .001
ADHD-EF Index	14.7	4.8	22.6	6.7	390.32	< .001
EF Symptom Count	6.9	12.5	29.2	21.0	426.02	< .001
EF Summary Score—Short Form	31.7	10.2	48.4	14.0	386.53	< .001
EF Symptom Count—Short Form	2.2	3.7	8.8	6.2	418.51	< .001

Note. F, results for the *F*-test; *p*, probability value for the *F*-test if ≤ .05; Self-Organization, Self-Organization/Problem Solving subscale; Self-Reg. of Emotion, Self-Regulation of Emotion subscale.

and were reported to be impaired in a major life activity. As stated in Chapter 4, this was the approach taken to establish the presence of ADHD in the sample so as to develop the ADHD-EF Index item list for the BDEFS-CA. There were 125 children in the original sample meeting these criteria. They were compared against the remainder of the sample (N= 1,797). The resulting differences were even larger than those in Table 7.3 and are shown in Table 7.4. All were significant, often averaging more than 2 *SD*s, which suggests minimal overlap in the distributions of scores for these two groups. The differences for the five BDEFS-CA subscales are also graphically portrayed in Figure 7.1, in which it is clearly evident that differences between the groups were substantial. Not only is all of this evidence for the validity of the BDEFS-CA, but it once again supports the conclusion that ADHD is very likely a developmental disorder of EF as theorized.

Speech and Language Disorders

Parents in the original sample indicated whether or not their children had been previously diagnosed by a professional as having a speech or language disorder (SLD). Although such indirect reports from parents are not the most rigorous approach to identifying children with SLD, this approach can still serve as a useful proxy for identifying children who are at least likely to have such disorders. Obviously, further research on children who were better screened and diagnosed directly by researchers would be the next logical step in such validation of the BDEFS-CA. But for the time being, this proxy method can provide some initial indication of validity. This problem of the limits of parent-reported diagnoses of their children occurs here for each of the diagnoses, and so it is not discussed again under each diagnosis.

TABLE 7.4. BDEFS-CA Long and Short Form Scores for Children in the Entire Sample Meeting Research Diagnostic Criteria for ADHD and the Sample Remainder

	No ADHD (N = 1,797)		ADHD (N = 125)			
Subscale	Mean	*SD*	Mean	*SD*	*F*	*p*
Self-Management to Time	22.4	7.5	41.1	7.6	725.15	< .001
Self-Organization	18.5	5.8	35.5	11.0	862.93	< .001
Self-Restraint	20.0	6.7	39.7	9.0	955.54	< .001
Self-Motivation	21.7	7.8	44.3	8.0	972.08	< .001
Self-Reg. of Emotion	24.1	8.8	47.6	12.6	777.30	< .001
Total EF Summary Score	106.7	31.0	208.3	36.6	1220.85	< .001
ADHD-EF Index	14.5	4.2	28.6	5.3	1279.26	< .001
EF Symptom Count	6.2	10.3	48.3	15.0	1799.80	< .001
EF Summary Score—Short Form	31.3	9.1	60.3	10.8	1157.69	< .001
EF Symptom Count—Short Form	2.0	3.2	14.1	4.5	1579.86	< .001

Note. F, results for the *F*-test; *p*, probability value for the *F*-test if ≤ .05; Self-Organization, Self-Organization/Problem Solving subscale; Self-Reg. of Emotion, Self-Regulation of Emotion subscale.

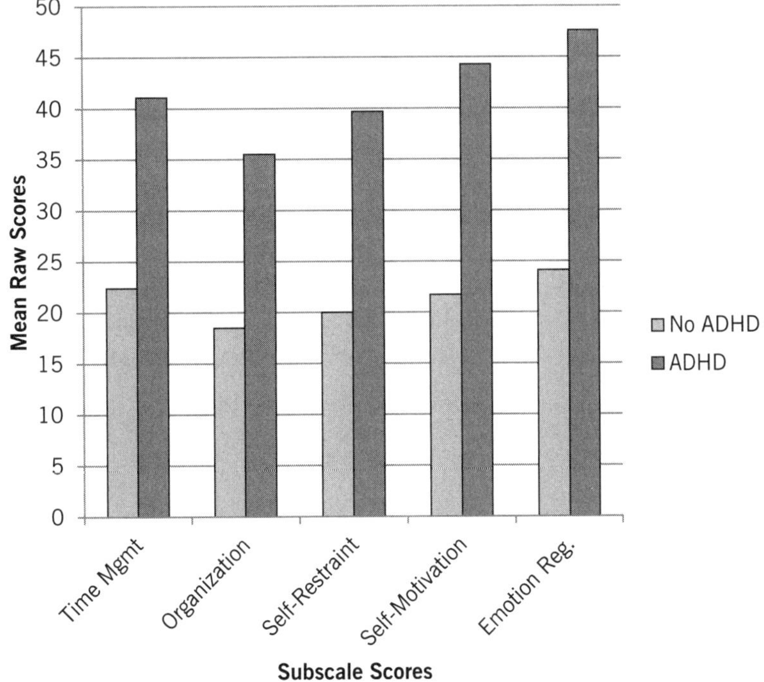

FIGURE 7.1. Raw scores for the BDEFS-CA subscales for children meeting research diagnostic criteria for ADHD compared with the remainder of the entire sample. Time Mgmt, Self-Management to Time subcale; Organization, Self-Organization/Problem Solving subscale; Emotion Reg., Self-Regulation of Emotion subscale.

Research indicates that a major EF component is verbal working memory and self-speech (see Chapter 1); language would be expected to be essential for normal development of this component (Gruber & Goschke, 2003). Indeed, the theory of EF on which this scale is based argues that verbal working memory is largely if not entirely based on self-directed and internalized self-speech and that such self-speech is often used for self-regulation, organization, and problem solving (Barkley, 1997a, 1997c, 2012b). As such, deficits in SLD would cascade into self-directed speech and verbal self-regulation and have some adverse impact on most components of EF to which language is related. Thus, children with SLD might be expected to have more deficits in EF than would children without such disorders but not as severely or pervasively as those with ADHD. For this manual, children in the original sample whose parents reported that they had a professional diagnosis of SLD ($N = 96$) were compared with the remainder of the sample ($N = 1{,}826$). Significant differences were evident on all 10 of the BDEFS-CA scores.

But children with both speech sound disorders and specific language impairments may have significantly greater likelihood of having ADHD, ranging from 16 to 66% (McGrath et al., 2008). This is especially so for the inattentive type of ADHD, given a greater association of such SLD with DSM-IV inattentive symptoms (McGrath et al., 2008). Therefore, any group differences in EF deficits between children with SLD and other children found previously might be a result of this comorbidity with ADHD. To control for this possibility, the group comparisons were repeated between the SLD group ($N = 72$) and nonimpaired children ($N = 1{,}725$), this time removing any children who met the preceding research criteria for ADHD ($N = 125$) from both groups. The results are shown in Table 7.5. The differences between groups are of a considerably smaller magnitude than was seen for the ADHD comparisons, which would be expected from hypothesizing a lesser impact

TABLE 7.5. BDEFS-CA Long and Short Form Scores for Children with and without a Professional Diagnosis of Speech or Language Delay (without ADHD)

	No delay ($N = 1{,}725$)		Language delayed ($N = 72$)			
Subscale	Mean	*SD*	Mean	*SD*	*F*	*p*
Self-Management to Time	22.3	7.5	24.1	6.4	3.94	.047
Self-Organization	18.3	5.5	23.1	9.3	49.50	< .001
Self-Restraint	19.9	6.7	21.3	6.8	2.65	NS
Self-Motivation	21.6	7.8	24.8	8.3	11.77	< .001
Self-Reg. of Emotion	24.0	8.8	26.5	9.8	5.84	.016
Total EF Summary Score	106.1	30.8	119.9	33.6	13.62	< .001
ADHD-EF Index	14.4	4.1	17.0	5.2	26.22	< .001
EF Symptom Count	6.0	10.2	10.8	12.8	14.65	< .001
EF Summary Score—Short Form	31.2	9.0	34.9	9.5	11.86	< .001
EF Symptom Count—Short Form	2.0	3.2	3.2	3.6	11.14	< .001

Note. F, results for the *F*-test; *p*, probability value for the *F*-test if ≤ .05; NS, nonsignificant; Self-Organization, Self-Organization/Problem Solving subscale; Self-Reg. of Emotion, Self-Regulation of Emotion subscale.

of SLD on EF, as discussed. All but one of the comparisons remained significant. The exception was the Self-Restraint (Inhibition) scale, suggesting that children with SLD are not characterized by such inhibitory deficits that are known to be an inherent component of ADHD (Barkley, 1997a, 1997c). SLD is not a disorder of inhibition, whereas ADHD is thought to have poor inhibition as one of its core components (American Psychiatric Association, 2000; Barkley, 1997a, 1997c).

However, this dataset also offers the opportunity to study parent ratings of EF deficits in children with SLD who are and are not comorbid for ADHD to examine whether there are unique patterns associated with one disorder relative to the other. In the next comparison, children with only SLD ($N = 72$) were compared with children having only ADHD (by the research criteria noted earlier; $N = 101$) and with those having both disorders (SLD + ADHD; $N = 24$). All three groups were compared with the remainder of the sample ($N = 1{,}725$). These comparisons were done with the five subscales of the BDEFS-CA in order to identify disorder-specific patterns in parent-rated EF deficits. The results appear in Figure 7.2. The omnibus ANOVAs were all significant (all p's < .001). Pairwise comparisons indicated that children with SLD + ADHD were significantly worse on the Self-Management

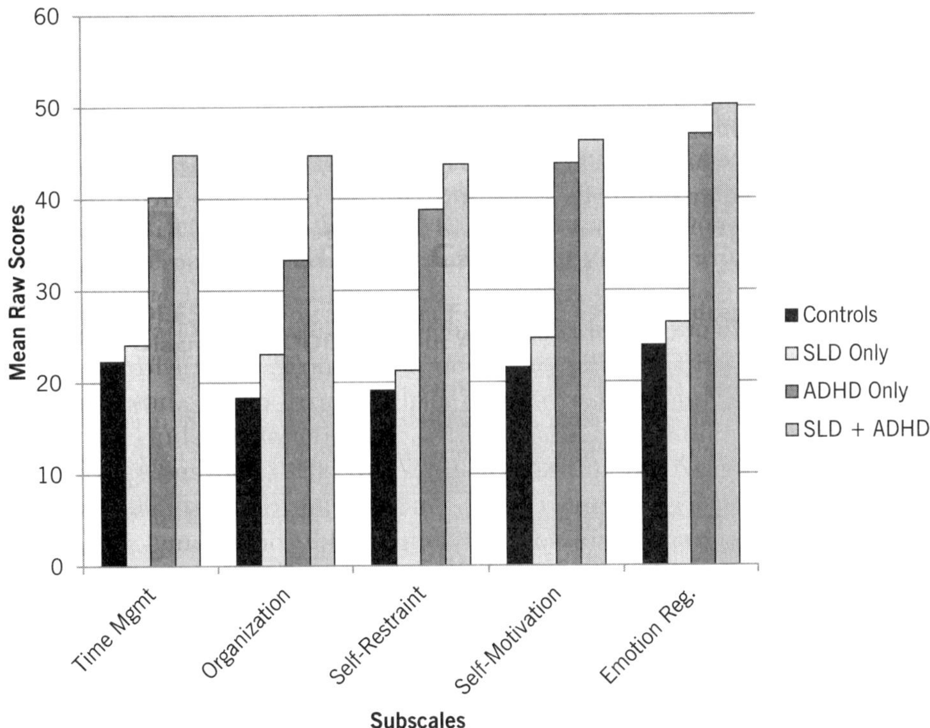

FIGURE 7.2. Raw scores for the BDEFS-CA subscales for children who had received a professional diagnosis of speech or language disorders (SLD) only, those having a research diagnosis of ADHD only, those with both disorders (SLD + ADHD), and the remainder of the sample (controls). Time Mgmt, Self-Management to Time subscale; Organization, Self-Organization/Problem Solving subscale; Emotion Reg., Self-Regulation of Emotion subscale.

to Time scale than all other groups. Those with ADHD only were also more deficient than the SLD-only and control groups, which did not differ from each other. Problems with time management are clearly not associated with SLD alone but are uniquely associated with ADHD, yet they are worse when the two disorders coexist. The pattern for the Self-Organization/Problem Solving subscale was somewhat different in that all groups were significantly different from the control group and from each other. They fell into a sequence based on severity of deficits such that SLD + ADHD > ADHD only > SLD only > controls. This suggests that both disorders have an adverse affect on this EF domain, though ADHD does so more adversely than does SLD, and that their effects are additive. Results for the Self-Restraint subscale were the same as for the time management dimension in that only the two groups with ADHD differed from the controls. Yet they also differed from each other in that SLD + ADHD was more deficient than ADHD only. The SLD-only group did not differ from the controls. Again this suggests that problems with Self-Restraint, just as with Self-Management to Time, are relatively specific to ADHD. Yet they can be somewhat worsened when it is comorbid with SLD. The pattern for the Self-Motivation scale was unique and differed from the preceding. The comorbid SLD + ADHD group and the ADHD group did not differ from each other, yet both differed from the SLD-only and control groups. Thus ADHD produces the most severe impact on this domain of EF whether or not it is comorbid with SLD. But the SLD-only group scored significantly worse than the controls even if not as deviant in this domain as the two ADHD groups. On the Self-Regulation of Emotion subscale, the results showed that it is ADHD that solely affects this dimension in that both ADHD groups scored significantly worse than the SLD-only and control groups who did not differ from each other.

To summarize, ADHD produces substantial and pervasive deficits across all five subscales of the BDEFS-CA, as noted earlier. In contrast, SLD alone is not associated with deficits in Self-Management to Time, Self-Restraint, or Self-Regulation of Emotion. But SLD is associated with some difficulties with Self-Organization/Problem Solving, as well as Self-Motivation, though not as severe as those associated with ADHD. Such findings make some sense when one considers the importance of language to internal or self-speech and to verbal working memory described earlier. Such self-directed speech would be important for performance in these two domains of EF in daily life (Barkley, 1997a, 2012b). This is also precisely the sort of evidence that provides substantial support for the criterion validity of the BDEFS-CA. It is relatively easy to show differences between disordered groups of children and normal samples on such a measure given that many disorders can interfere with EF, especially as it is used in daily life activities. It is a more difficult test of a measure to show that it can detect relatively unique patterns of EF deficits associated with different disorders. The BDEFS-CA can do so.

Delayed Motor Development or Coordination

Children with delayed motor development and coordination, also known as developmental coordination disorder (DCD), have been shown to have some cognitive deficits, specifically deficient visual–spatial reasoning, beyond just difficulties with motor tasks (Loh, Piek, & Barrett, 2011; Piek, Dyck, Francis, & Conwell, 2007).

Because visual–spatial ability is also linked to the EF component of nonverbal working memory, it is likely that children with DCD may have some EF deficits, particularly in this type of working memory (Piek et al., 2007). Children with a professional diagnosis of DCD ($N = 63$) were compared with those without such a diagnosis ($N = 1,859$) on the 10 BDEFS-CA, scores and all were significant (all p's < .001). However, comparisons of children with and without DCD are complicated by the high comorbidity of DCD with ADHD, which can range from 13 to 50% or more of such cases (Barkley, 2006; Kaplan, Crawford, Cantell, Kooistra, & Dewey, 2006; Piek et al., 2007). Once again, children with ADHD were removed from the groups of children with and without DCD so that comparisons could be made between these two groups without being confounded with cases of ADHD that are likely to have substantial deficits in EF. All comparisons remained significant (all p's < .003) and are shown in Table 7.6.

Again, of greater interest and importance to scale validity is the presence of any distinct patterns between different disorders that may sometimes be comorbid. To examine this possibility, children with DCD only ($N = 40$) were compared with those with ADHD only ($N = 102$) and with those with both disorders (DCD + ADHD; $N = 23$). All were compared with the remaining control children. The results are shown in Figure 7.3 for the five subscale scores. The omnibus ANOVAs were all significant (all p's < .001). The pattern was the same for four of the five scales. On those four scales, both groups with ADHD had significantly greater EF deficits than the DCD-only and control groups yet did not differ from each other. Even so, the DCD-only group also had more such problems than controls even if not to the degree seen in the two ADHD groups. But on the Self-Organization/Problem Solving subscale, the groups all differed from each other and in the sequence

TABLE 7.6. BDEFS-CA Long and Short Form Scores for Children with and without a Professional Diagnosis of DCD (without ADHD)

	No DCD (no ADHD) (N = 1,757)		DCD (no ADHD) (N = 40)			
Subscale	Mean	*SD*	Mean	*SD*	*F*	*p*
Self-Management to Time	22.3	7.5	25.9	6.7	9.10	.003
Self-Organization	18.3	5.5	25.9	11.1	68.66	< .001
Self-Restraint	19.9	6.7	23.1	7.6	8.85	.003
Self-Motivation	21.6	7.8	26.8	8.0	17.60	< .001
Self-Reg. of Emotion	24.0	8.8	28.1	9.1	8.79	.003
Total EF Summary Score	106.2	30.8	129.9	33.4	23.17	< .001
ADHD-EF Index	14.4	4.1	18.3	5.5	33.83	< .001
EF Symptom Count	6.0	10.2	13.5	12.4	20.59	< .001
EF Summary Score—Short Form	31.2	9.0	37.1	9.5	16.57	< .001
EF Symptom Count—Short Form	2.0	3.2	3.9	3.6	14.23	< .001

Note. DCD, developmental coordination disorder; F, results for the F-test; p, probability value for the F-test if ≤ .05; Self-Organization, Self-Organization/Problem Solving subscale; Self-Reg. of Emotion, Self-Regulation of Emotion subscale.

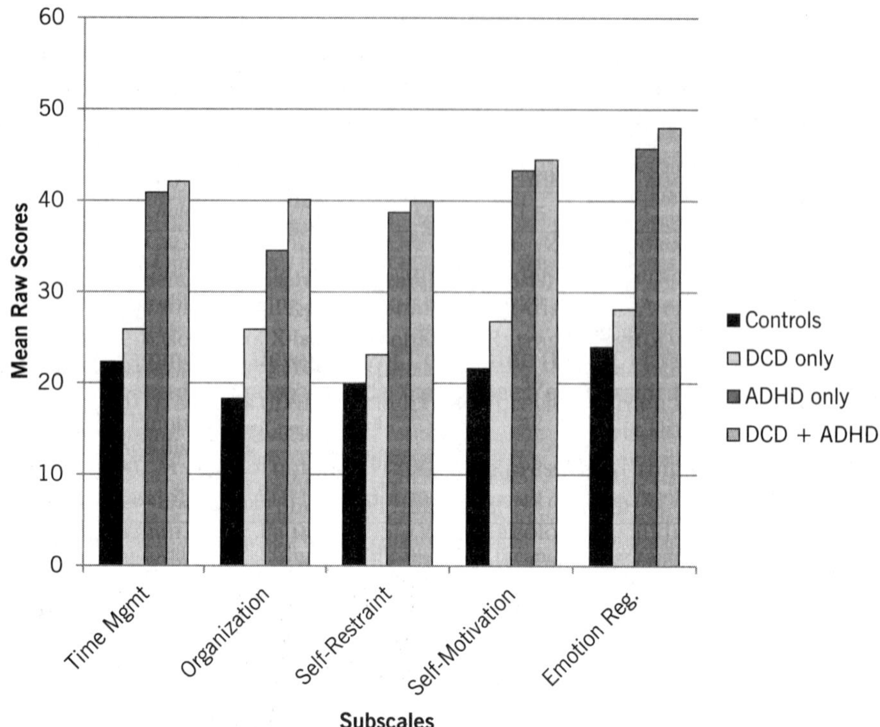

FIGURE 7.3. Raw scores for the BDEFS-CA subscales for children who had received a professional diagnosis of motor delay or motor coordination difficulties (DCD) alone, ADHD alone, and both disorders (DCD + ADHD) compared with the remainder of the entire sample. Time Mgmt, Self-Management to Time subscale; Organization, Self-Organization/Problem-Solving subscale; Emotion Reg., Self-Regulation of Emotion subscale.

of the severity of their deficits with DCD + ADHD > ADHD only > DCD only > controls. Here, both disorders are contributing to difficulties with Self-Organization/Problem Solving, though ADHD contributes more than does DCD. The difficulties each disorder contributes to this domain are additive when in the comorbid state. Here again one also finds strong evidence for the validity of the BDEFS-CA apart from the importance of such findings for understanding the impact of DCD and ADHD on EF in children's daily life activities.

Further evidence for the validity of the BDEFS-CA in detecting differential patterns of EF impairments in daily life would come from comparing children with DCD only with those with SLD and those having both disorders. In view of the previous discussion of each disorder, they would arise from different neurodevelopmental mechanisms in the brain. Yet they may have some overlap with each other in that the expressive speech center is directly related to the oral–vocal motor networks of the frontal cortex, which is clearly a part of the larger motor system of that brain region. One could anticipate that these disorders would have different patterns of impact on EF in daily life, even though they should be far less severe than those deficits associated with ADHD. In fact, given the overlap of both disorders with ADHD, its presence would contaminate or confound the results, especially if

ADHD were more differentially associated with one disorder than the other. Consequently children with ADHD were removed from the following comparisons. There were 61 children in the sample who had been diagnosed as having SLD only (but not ADHD or DCD), 29 who had been diagnosed with DCD only (but not ADHD or SLD), and 11 who had comorbid DCD + SLD (but not ADHD). The omnibus ANOVAs were all significant for the five subscales of the BDEFS-CA (all p's < .01). The results are shown in Figure 7.4 and clearly show a milder impact of these disorders on EF ratings than was the case for ADHD. Yet a differential pattern can still be detected between the disorders through the pairwise contrasts. On three subscales, the groups did not differ from each other (Self-Management to Time, Self-Restraint, and Self-Regulation of Emotion). This makes perfect sense given that neither disorder is believed to affect EF components that would be crucial to these EF dimensions in daily life. But both disorders did have a detrimental, if mild, impact on Self-Organization/Problem Solving, with the comorbid group having the greatest EF problems in this domain, greater than the SLD-only or DCD-only cases. The latter groups did not differ from each other, but both differed from the controls in having higher EF deficit scores. This finding intimates that the two disorders may have distinct yet comparable effects on this domain of EF and, when

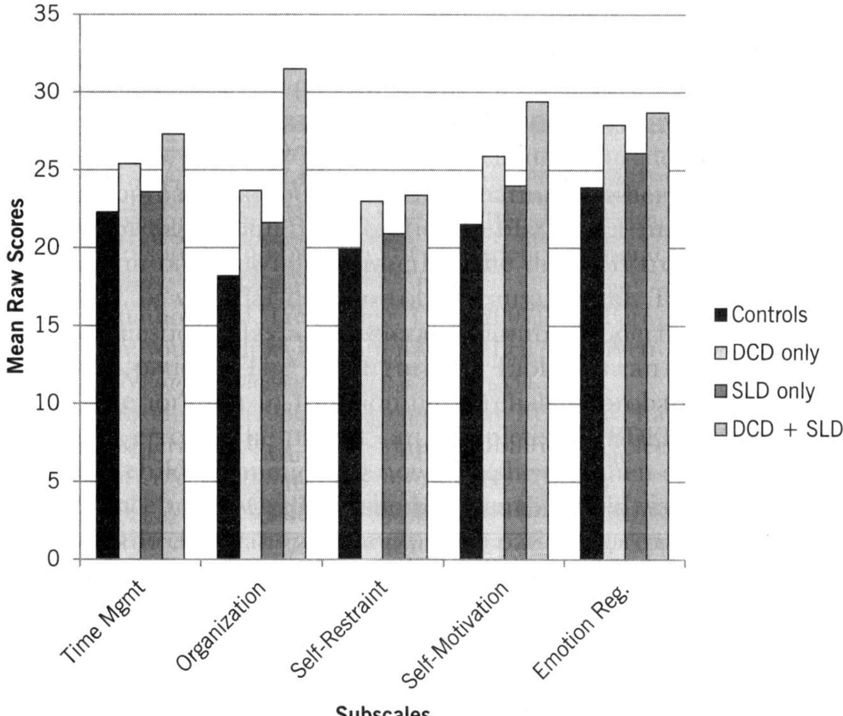

FIGURE 7.4. Raw scores for the BDEFS-CA subscales for children who had received a professional diagnosis of DCD alone, SLD alone, and both disorders (DCD + SLD) compared with the remainder of the entire sample after removal of all ADHD cases. Time Mgmt, Self-Management to Time subscale; Organization, Self-Organization/Problem Solving subscale; Emotion Reg., Self-Regulation of Emotion subscale.

combined, may cause an additive result of greater deficits for the comorbid group. For the Self-Motivation domain, SLD did not differ from the control group. Only the comorbid DCD + SLD group had higher scores than those in the SLD-only and control groups. The DCD-only group fell between the comorbid and the other groups, not differing from any of them. This suggests that it is DCD that has the greater impact on Self-Motivation, an effect made worse when it is comorbid with SLD. This is yet more evidence for the validity of the BDEFS-CA to differentiate among disorders in their patterns of deficits.

Developmental Delay/Mental Retardation

The original sample contained 22 children whose parents reported that they had been diagnosed by a professional as having developmental delay/mental retardation (DD/MR). Deficits in EF would be expected in individuals having such a generalized delay in development, and indeed reviews indicate that regardless of etiology, DD/MR is typically associated with deficits in attention, short-term or working memory, and sequential processing (Pulsifer, 1996). More specific deficits in other EF components can be found in cases in which the etiology of the MR is known, as in genetic disorders such as Down syndrome or in acquired cases such as may be due to fetal alcohol syndrome (FAS; Pulsifer, 1996) or Williams syndrome (Mervis & John, 2010). For instance, in fragile X syndrome, difficulties with EF as assessed on psychometric tests are commonly found but are related to the level of general intellectual delay. In contrast, specific problems with using intentions to guide or regulate behavior were associated with this form of DD/MR that were independent of generalized cognitive delay (Loesch et al., 2003). Another example of more specific EF deficits with specific etiologies of DD/MR can be seen in children exposed to heavy alcohol use, including those meeting criteria for FAS. Research suggests that such children have their greatest difficulties with the EF components of planning and response inhibition, although other components may also be affected, such as abstract thinking and flexibility (Mattson, Goodman, Caine, Delis, & Riley, 2006), and that meeting criteria for FAS made no difference in these results in comparison with control-group children. Deficits on parent ratings of EF (BRIEF) have also been found in children with prenatal alcohol exposure, again without regard to whether or not the children met criteria for FAS (Schonfeld, Paley, Frankel, & O'Connor, 2006). So there is very good reason to suspect that deficits in EF in daily life activities as reflected on the BDEFS-CA would be associated with DD/MR.

To explore this possibility, the 22 children carrying a professional diagnosis of DD/MR according to parent-report were compared with the remainder of the sample (1,900). All comparisons were significant (all p's $< .001$). But 13 of these children also met the research criteria for ADHD, which is not an uncommon rate of comorbid ADHD within samples of children with DD/MR. Even when these cases were removed, the differences between those with DD/MR (without ADHD; N = 12) and the remainder ($N = 1,785$) remained significant (all p's $\leq .01$ except for Self-Management to Time, $p = .025$). These differences were significant despite the very low power of the comparison due to the very small DD/MR sample. Those results are shown in Table 7.7.

TABLE 7.7. BDEFS-CA Long and Short Form Scores for Children with and without a Professional Diagnosis of DD/MR (without ADHD)

	No DD/MR (no ADHD) (N= 1,788)		DD/MR (no ADHD) (N= 9)			
Subscale	Mean	*SD*	Mean	*SD*	*F*	*p*
Self-Management to Time	22.4	7.5	28.0	7.1	5.02	.025
Self-Organization	18.4	5.6	34.0	14.0	67.07	< .001
Self-Restraint	20.0	6.7	25.4	8.3	5.93	.015
Self-Motivation	21.7	7.8	31.2	8.5	13.44	< .001
Self-Reg. of Emotion	24.0	8.8	32.1	8.9	7.54	.006
Total EF Summary Score	106.5	30.9	150.8	35.9	18.48	< .001
ADHD-EF Index	14.5	4.1	23.3	6.4	40.92	< .001
EF Symptom Count	6.1	10.3	22.9	12.9	23.74	< .001
EF Summary Score—Short Form	31.3	9.0	42.2	10.2	13.06	< .001
EF Symptom Count—Short Form	2.0	3.2	6.1	3.5	14.93	< .001

Note. DD/MR, developmental delay/mental retardation; F = results for the F-test; p = probability value for the F-test if ≤ .05; Self-Organization, Self-Organization/Problem Solving subscale; Self-Reg. of Emotion, Self-Regulation of Emotion subscale.

Seizure Disorders or Epilepsy

In the original sample, parents of 14 children reported that their children were professionally diagnosed with a seizure disorder or epilepsy. Deficits in EF on psychometric tests have been demonstrated in children with temporal lobe epilepsy (TLE), with earlier onset of seizures being associated with greater such deficits (Black et al., 2010). EF deficits might be expected to vary in such children as a function of the brain region involved in generating the seizure disorder. For instance, comparisons of children with frontal lobe epilepsy with those with TLE suggest that the former have more problems with EF and impulse control, whereas the latter are more likely to show deficits in memory (Culhane-Shelburne, Chapieski, Hiscock, & Glaze, 2002). That study also found that the extent of EF deficits in both groups of children was directly related to their degree of difficulties in adaptive functioning. We were not able to make such a distinction among the sources of the seizures with the children in the original sample who had diagnoses of epilepsy. Yet there was good reason given the preceding findings to believe that such children would be more likely to have deficits on the BDEFS-CA than children without such disorders. The 14 children with diagnoses of a seizure disorder were compared with the remainder of the sample (N = 1,908) on all 10 BDEFS-CA scores, and all were significant (all p's < .001). Just two of the children in the seizure disorder group had diagnoses of ADHD, and so they were not removed from the group for any further comparisons given the already low power of the sample having seizure disorders. The results are shown in Table 7.8. As that table shows, not all comparisons were significant. The group with the seizure disorders differed on most scales except for the Self-Restraint and Self-Regulation of Emotion subscales. In view of the higher

TABLE 7.8. BDEFS-CA Long and Short Form Scores for Children with and without a Professional Diagnosis of Seizure Disorder or Epilepsy (without ADHD)

	No seizure disorder (no ADHD) (N= 1,785)		Seizure disorder (no ADHD) (N= 12)			
Subscale	Mean	*SD*	Mean	*SD*	*F*	*p*
Self-Management to Time	23.6	8.8	29.9	12.2	5.10	.024
Self-Organization	19.5	7.4	30.2	12.8	28.30	< .001
Self-Restraint	21.2	8.4	25.6	12.4	3.64	NS
Self-Motivation	23.1	9.6	29.0	12.0	5.17	.023
Self-Reg. of Emotion	25.6	10.8	29.8	13.8	2.19	NS
Total EF Summary Score	113.1	40.0	143.6	57.6	8.03	.005
ADHD-EF Index	15.4	5.5	20.6	8.4	12.61	< .001
EF Symptom Count	8.8	14.8	22.3	20.7	11.32	.001
EF Summary Score—Short Form	33.2	11.6	40.3	16.4	5.19	.023
EF Symptom Count—Short Form	2.8	4.4	5.7	6.2	6.04	.014

Note. F, results for the *F*-test; *p*, probability value for the *F*-test if ≤ .05; NS, nonsignificant; Self-Organization, Self-Organization/Problem Solving subscale; Self-Reg. of Emotion, Self-Regulation of Emotion subscale.

mean scores on even these scales, it is likely that with a larger sample of children with seizure disorders even these comparisons might have been significant.

Tic Disorders or Tourette Syndrome

Simple or transient tics are a common occurrence in children, being found in 7–21% of general population samples of children (Clements, Lee, & Barclay, 1988; Khalifa & Knorring, 2007; Kurlan et al., 2002), with nearly 7% of children having experienced some form of tic in the preceding year (Khalifa & Knorring, 2007). Most such simple tics tend to remit within 4 years of onset (Leckman, 2004; Spencer et al., 1999). Such occurrences rarely result in a professional diagnosis of a disorder. Far less common are children with multiple tics that often do lead to a diagnosis of a chronic or multiple tic disorder (TD) or Tourette syndrome (TS). TS occurs in approximately 0.1–6 individuals per 1,000, or 0.01–0.60% (Khalifa & Knorring, 2007; Singer & Walkup, 1991). In the present sample, parents reported a professional diagnosis of TD/TS in 11 children, or 0.5% of our sample, consistent with that found in other studies using more rigorous ascertainment of the disorder. Early studies typically found significant deficits on psychometric tests of EF in children with TD/TS (Leckman, 2004). So there was some reason to believe that such children would also display deficits on parent ratings of EF. To test this idea, the children in the present sample having TD/TS were compared with those without tics on all 10 scores from the BDEFS-CA. All of the differences were significant and fairly substantial (all *p*'s < .001). But there is a considerably higher incidence of ADHD (and obsessive–compulsive disorder) in children with TD/TS (typically

30–50% or more) (Banaschewski, Neale, Rothenberger, & Roessner, 2007; Kurlan et al., 2002; Leckman, 2004) than the base rates for either disorder would predict. Again, the coexistence of ADHD with TD/TS could be the basis for these differences in EF ratings. TD/TS are also overrepresented in ADHD, being present in up to 20%, perhaps more, of those cases (Banaschewski et al., 2007; Barkley, 2006; Spencer et al., 1999). Indeed, when cases of TD/TS are separated on the basis of comorbidity with ADHD, EF deficits on tests are diminished considerably; they may be found only on tests of attention or motor control or are, more often, exclusively associated only with those children having ADHD (Groot, Yeates, Baker, & Bornstein, 1997; Harris et al., 1995; Roessner, Becker, Banaschewski, & Rothenberger, 2007). This appears to be the case with parent ratings of EF deficits as well. Deficits have been found on all scales of the BRIEF in individuals with ADHD or ADHD with TS, but not in cases with TS alone (Mahone et al., 2002).

In this sample, just 3 of the 11 children professionally diagnosed with TD/TS also met criteria for a diagnosis of ADHD (27%). They were therefore removed from the sample, and the scores were reanalyzed. Those results are shown in Table 7.9 and were essentially the same as the initial analyses, though the mean differences were diminished somewhat. All but one of the scores remained significant, the exception being the Self-Management to Time scale ($p = .083$). Again, despite substantially limited power to detect effects due to the very small sample size of TD/TS cases, the results suggest that problems with managing oneself relative to time and deadlines is fairly specific to cases of TD/TS without ADHD, whereas other EF deficits in daily life activities may be associated with TD/TS alone, even if not evident on psychometric testing.

TABLE 7.9. BDEFS-CA Long and Short Form Scores for Children with and without a Professional Diagnosis of TD/TS (without ADHD)

	No TD/TS (no ADHD) (N = 1,789)		TD/TS (no ADHD) (N = 8)			
Subscale	Mean	*SD*	Mean	*SD*	*F*	*p*
Self-Management to Time	22.4	7.5	27.0	4.9	2.99	NS
Self-Organization	18.5	5.8	23.7	5.4	6.60	.010
Self-Restraint	20.0	6.7	26.7	7.0	8.10	.004
Self-Motivation	21.7	7.8	27.2	4.6	4.03	.045
Self-Reg. of Emotion	24.0	8.8	36.5	9.1	16.09	< .001
Total EF Summary Score	106.5	31.0	141.2	21.8	10.00	.002
ADHD-EF Index	14.5	4.2	18.7	3.1	8.21	.004
EF Symptom Count	6.2	10.3	16.4	10.7	7.76	.005
EF Summary Score—Short Form	31.3	9.1	40.4	5.2	7.97	.005
EF Symptom Count—Short Form	2.0	3.2	4.5	2.5	4.84	.028

Note. TD/TS, tic disorder/Tourette syndrome; F = results for the F-test; p = probability value for the F-test if ≤ .05; NS, nonsignificant; Self-Organization, Self-Organization/Problem Solving subscale; Self-Reg. of Emotion, Self-Regulation of Emotion subscale.

Autism Spectrum Disorders

Studies suggest that autism spectrum disorders (ASD) occur in approximately 0.6–1.0% of the child and adolescent population (Simonoff et al., 2008). Numerous studies have demonstrated significant deficits in EF both on psychometric tests (Guerts, Verte, Oosterlaan, Roeyers, & Sergeant, 2004; Pennington & Ozonoff, 1996; Rogers, 1998; Semrud-Clikeman, Walkowiak, Wilkinson, & Butcher, 2010) and on parent ratings of EF deficits (Gilotty et al., 2002; Gioia, Isquith, Kenworthy, & Barton, 2002; Semrud-Clikeman et al., 2010; Zandt et al., 2009) in children with ASD, though this is not always the case for psychometric tests of EF (Griffith, Pennington, Wehner, & Rogers, 2003; Zandt et al., 2009). Again, this is usually because low or no significant relationships exist between EF tests and EF ratings (Zandt et al., 2009). On tests, ASD may be associated with a broad spectrum of deficits, but most difficulties are in planning, strategy formation and initiation, and sometimes in verbal working memory rather than inhibition, interference control (resistance to distraction), or verbal fluency (Corbett, Constantine, Hendren, Rocke, & Ozonoff, 2009; Guerts et al., 2004; Pennington & Ozonoff, 1996). In contrast, children with ADHD relative to those with ASD often have more difficulties on tasks assessing response inhibition and working memory, especially the nonverbal component (Guerts et al., 2004; Pennington & Ozonoff, 1996; Semrud-Clikeman et al., 2010). Comparisons of these two groups on parental ratings of EF likewise show that both groups manifest pervasive EF deficits relative to control-group children (Gioia et al., 2002; Semrud-Clikeman et al., 2010), with both having especially high elevations on behavioral regulation and emotional control. In one study the degree of both ADHD and ASD symptoms was directly linked to elevations on both factors of the BRIEF (Metacognition and Behavioral Regulation; Semrud-Clikeman et al., 2010). In another study, children with ASD showed more difficulties with metacognition (flexibility) relative to children with other disorders, such as ADHD, reading disorders, or TBI (Gioia et al., 2002), whereas children with ADHD showed more serious problems with inhibitory deficits compared with these other groups.

In the present sample, parents of 36 children (1.8%) reported that their children had received professional diagnoses of autism, ASD, or Asperger syndrome. These children composed the ASD group and were compared with the remainder of the sample (N = 1,886) on all 10 BDEFS-CA scores. All comparisons were significant (all p's < .001). Differences between these groups were substantial, rivaling those magnitudes seen previously in the comparisons involving children with ADHD and implying that substantial and pervasive difficulties in all EF domains in daily life are associated with ASD.

However, ADHD is the second most common comorbid disorder associated with ASD after social anxiety disorder (Simonoff et al., 2008). Studies suggest that 28–53% of children with ASD may have ADHD (Simonoff et al., 2008; Sinzig, Walter, & Doepfner, 2009). The rate of comorbidity between ADHD and ASD in the present ASD sample was 47% (17 of 36), consistent with prior studies. Likewise, children with ADHD often have significant elevations in ASD symptoms even if they do not qualify for a diagnosis of ASD (Mulligan et al., 2009; Reiersen, Constantino, Volk, & Todd, 2007). Interestingly, behavioral genetic studies of twins show that these two symptom dimensions have a high degree of shared familial genetic contribution between them (Mulligan et al., 2009). That contribution is also shared with the degree of conduct disorder, oppositional defiant disorder, and motor disorders. Thus, removing children with ADHD from such studies of EF ratings in children with ASD may remove some of the variance in EF that is actually due to ASD (the independent variable of interest) or that at least is the result of this shared underlying familial trait. Even so, the ADHD cases were removed from the ASD sample, and the analyses were recomputed. All analyses except Self-Management to Time remained significant, indicating that it is ADHD that is driving the group difference on that domain in children with ASD compared with control-group children. These results are shown in Table 7.10. This suggests that time management is not a special EF problem for children with ASD.

However, it would be more informative to study the resulting patterns of EF deficits for each disorder alone and their comorbidity. There were 17 children with ASD only, 108 with ADHD only, and 17 with both disorders (ASD + ADHD) for comparison with the remainder of the sample (N = 1,778). All omnibus ANOVAs were significant at $p < .001$, and the results are portrayed graphically in Figure 7.5. The pairwise contrasts were quite informative. For four of the five subscales, the two ADHD groups had significantly higher scores than did the ASD-only or control groups, with the two ADHD groups not differing from each other. This occurred on the subscales of Self-Management to Time, Self-Restraint, Self-Motivation, and Self-Regulation of Emotion. In the time management domain, the ASD-only and control groups did not differ. But in the other three subscales, the ASD group did show higher scores than the control group, though significantly below the two ADHD groups. All of this suggests that ADHD impairs EF in daily life activities more than does ASD. ASD does seem to have some mild adverse effects in some EF domains,

TABLE 7.10. BDEFS-CA Long and Short Form Scores for Children with and without a Professional Diagnosis of ASD without ADHD

	No ASD (no ADHD) (N = 1,778)		ASD (no ADHD) (N = 19)			
Subscale	Mean	*SD*	Mean	*SD*	*F*	*p*
Self-Management to Time	22.4	7.5	24.9	6.2	2.18	NS
Self-Organization	18.4	5.7	27.4	9.6	46.62	< .001
Self-Restraint	19.9	6.7	26.9	9.2	20.33	< .001
Self-Motivation	21.7	7.8	26.1	9.2	6.06	.014
Self-Reg. of Emotion	23.9	8.7	34.5	11.3	27.37	< .001
Total EF Summary Score	106.3	30.8	139.9	35.0	22.21	< .001
ADHD-EF Index	14.5	4.1	19.5	5.3	27.79	< .001
EF Symptom Count	6.1	10.2	18.0	14.0	25.20	< .001
EF Summary Score—Short Form	31.2	9.0	40.4	9.9	19.14	< .001
EF Symptom Count—Short Form	2.0	3.2	5.2	4.2	19.32	< .001

Note. ASD, autism spectrum disorder; F = results for the F-test; p = probability value for the F-test if ≤ .05; NS, nonsignificant; Self-Organization, Self-Organization/Problem Solving subscale; Self-Reg. of Emotion, Self-Regulation of Emotion subscale.

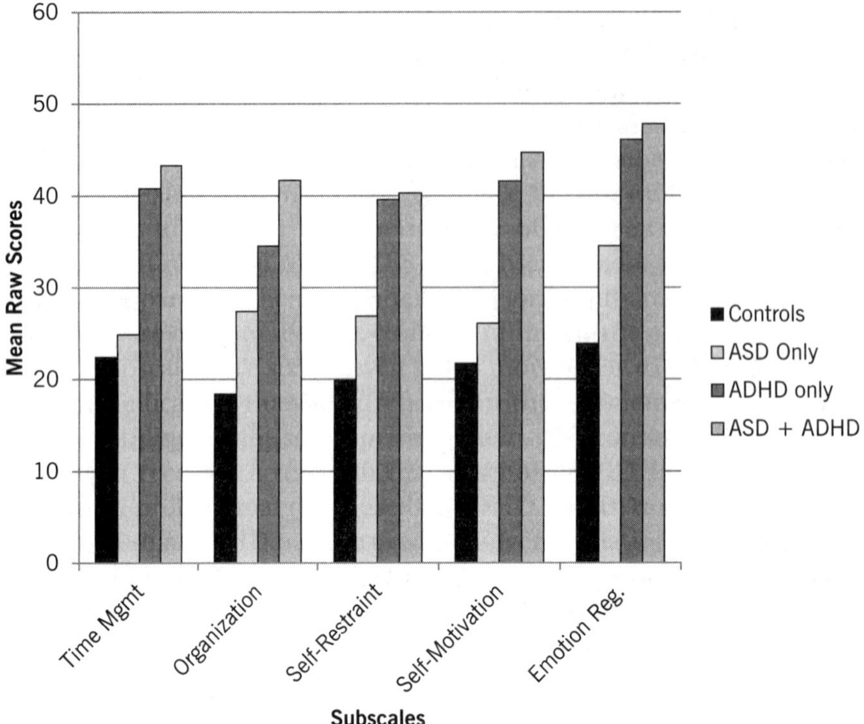

FIGURE 7.5. Raw scores for the BDEFS-CA subscales for children who had received a professional diagnosis of autism spectrum disorders (ASD) alone, ADHD alone, those with both disorders (ASD + ADHD), and the remainder of the sample (controls). Time Mgmt, Self-Management to Time subscale; Organization, Self-Organization/Problem Solving subscale; Emotion Reg., Self-Regulation of Emotion subscale.

nonetheless. Yet even then its contribution is not additive when the two disorders coexist, implying that its contribution when alone could be due to the coexistence of high but subclinical levels of ADHD symptoms in the ASD-only group. Given the shared familial genetic contribution to both disorders, this would not be surprising. The exception to this pattern was on the Self-Organization/Problem Solving subscale, on which all four groups differed from each other. Their order of diminishing severity was ASD + ADHD > ADHD only > ASD only > controls. Even this pattern still suggests that ADHD is a more impairing disorder in this EF domain than is ASD. The combination of the two has an additive effect, making the deficits even worse than occur in either disorder alone. Although these results are not directly comparable to those for the BRIEF, discussed earlier, they may be consistent given that the Metacognitive scale on the BRIEF contains the domains of organization and problem-solving items. Both studies show that ASD may have some specific effects in this domain. But ADHD produced more adverse effects on the Behavioral Regulation domain of the BRIEF in those studies. This would be expected given that the Behavior Regulation scale contains items pertaining to the Self-Restraint (Inhibition) and Emotional Self-Regulation dimensions of the BDEFS-CA. Again, such findings are not just scientifically informative but also clearly supportive of the validity of the BDEFS-CA in discriminating patterns among various learning, developmental, and psychiatric disorders.

ASD is known to have a significant association with SLD in view of the often impaired, if not bizarre, language development associated with ASD. Is the impact of ASD on EF due to its association with such language delays? This shows that yet another informative comparison is possible within this sample. It would also provide additional evidence for the validity of the BDEFS-CA in differentiating between various disorders that have some impact on EF. Both disorders are associated with ADHD. Therefore, cases of ADHD were initially removed from any comparisons between these disorders. There were 14 cases of ASD only (no ADHD or SLD), 67 cases of SLD only (no ADHD or ASD), and 5 cases of ASD + SLD, all of which were compared with the remainder of the sample (no ADHD; $N = 1{,}711$). Four of the five omnibus ANOVAs were significant at $p < .001$, whereas that for the Self-Management to Time scale was not significant. This suggests that neither disorder is associated with impairments in that EF domain separate from any overlap they have with ADHD; again, it is ADHD that is the disorder of time management. The comparisons for all the BDEFS-CA subscales are shown in Figure 7.6.

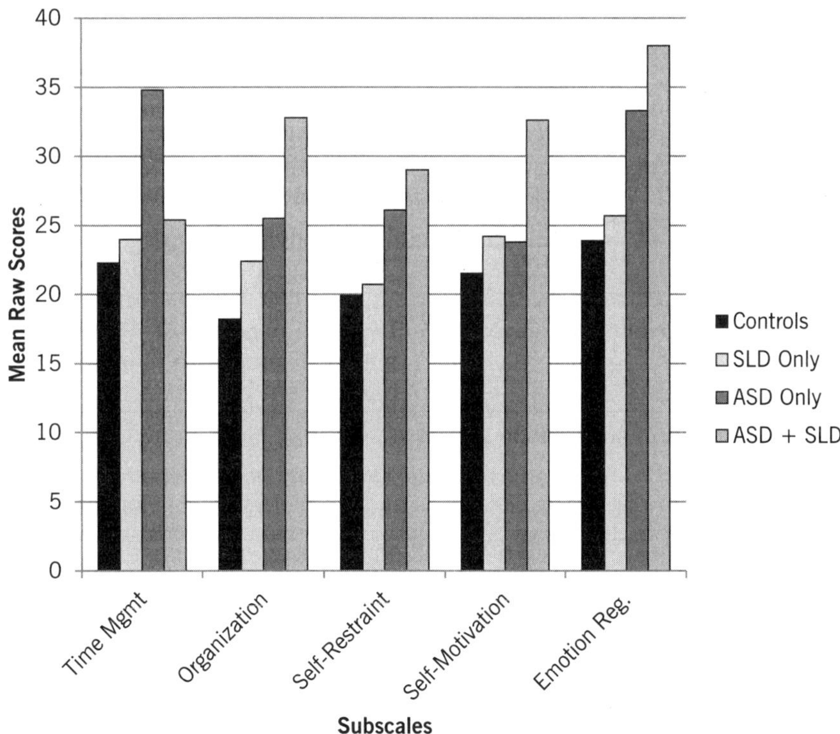

FIGURE 7.6. Raw scores for the BDEFS-CA subscales for children who had received a professional diagnosis of SLD alone, ASD alone, those with both disorders (ASD + SLD), and the remainder of the sample (controls) with all cases of ADHD removed from the groups. Time Mgmt, Self-Management to Time subscale; Organization, Self-Organization/Problem Solving subscale; Emotion Reg., Self-Regulation of Emotion subscale. ADHD = Attention Deficit Hyperactivity Disorder.

The pairwise comparisons showed that both the ASD-only and comorbid groups had higher scores on Self-Organization/Problem Solving than did control-group children, but the comorbid group scored significantly worse than the ASD-only group and worse than the SLD-only group, which did not differ from the control-group (or ASD-only) children. In this domain, ASD is the more impairing disorder, but comorbid SLD can accentuate those deficits. Both of the ASD groups had higher scores in the Self-Restraint domain than did the control or SLD-only groups. The two ASD groups were not different in this regard, and thus it is ASD that is linked more to problems with inhibition in daily life activities, not SLD. This same pattern was evident for the domain of Self-Regulation of Emotion, which makes sense given that no argument has been made that SLD disrupts this domain of EF. In contrast, a strong case has been made for ASD being likely to do so given that it has a strong association with anxiety, irritability, and emotional dysregulation more generally. In the domain of Self-Motivation, only the comorbid group differed from the other three groups, which did not differ from each other. Again, such comparisons involve small samples that limit the power to detect less than large or robust effect sizes; more research on this issue is warranted. Nevertheless, what distinct patterns did emerge here for ASD over SLD support the validity of the BDEFS-CA as a useful tool in differentiating the disorders.

Specific Learning Disabilities

Reading Disorders

Reading disorders (RD) occur in approximately 5–9% of children (Shaywitz, Shaywitz, Fletcher, & Escobar, 1990) and are known to encompass significant problems with language beyond just difficulties with reading. As a consequence, children with RD may also have difficulties with EF, particularly in verbal working memory tasks. But this linkage of RD or dyslexia to EF deficits is complicated by the high comorbidity between RD and ADHD (Germanò, Gagliano, & Curatolo, 2010), which often ranges from 15 to 30% of ADHD cases (Barkley, 2006; Del'Homme, Kim, Loo, Yang, & Smalley, 2007). Studies that have compared children with each disorder alone have shown that RD is linked to lexical decision impairments, whereas ADHD is not. Some studies found RD to be associated with difficulties on inhibitory tasks relative to children with ADHD alone, who have problems in both inhibition and nonverbal working memory tasks (Jong et al., 2009). Studies using parent ratings of EF have also found significant deficits in EF in daily life activities in children with RD compared with controls. But these deficits are often significantly milder than the more severe deficits in EF ratings associated with ADHD or ASD (Gioia et al., 2002). For this manual, comparisons were made between children with professional diagnoses of RD ($N = 77$) and the remainder ($N = 1{,}845$) on all BDEFS-CA scores, and all were significant ($p < .001$). But once again it was important to remove those children with ADHD from these comparisons. When this was done and the comparisons were repeated, all comparisons remained significant. The results are shown in Table 7.11. This result not only supports earlier findings that RD is associated with some EF deficits independent of its relationship to ADHD but also provides further evidence for the validity of the BDEFS-CA.

TABLE 7.11. BDEFS-CA Long and Short Form Scores for Children with and without a Professional Diagnosis of RD (without ADHD)

	No RD (no ADHD) (N = 1,743)		RD (no ADHD) (N = 54)			
Subscale	Mean	*SD*	Mean	*SD*	*F*	*p*
Self-Management to Time	22.3	7.5	26.3	7.0	15.27	< .001
Self-Organization	18.3	5.7	23.5	7.2	42.30	< .001
Self-Restraint	19.9	6.7	22.2	7.0	5.78	.016
Self-Motivation	21.5	7.7	27.2	8.1	27.79	< .001
Self-Reg. of Emotion	24.0	8.8	27.3	9.0	7.65	.006
Total EF Summary Score	106.1	30.9	126.5	29.8	22.99	< .001
ADHD-EF Index	14.4	4.1	17.6	4.4	30.33	< .001
EF Symptom Count	6.0	10.2	12.0	12.3	17.75	< .001
EF Summary Score—Short Form	31.2	9.0	37.1	8.2	22.57	< .001
EF Symptom Count—Short Form	2.0	3.2	3.7	3.7	16.60	< .001

Note. RD, reading disorder; *F*, results for the *F*-test; *p*, probability value for the *F*-test if ≤ .05; Self-Reg. of Emotion, Self-Regulation of Emotion subscale.

Even stronger evidence for such conclusions, however, comes once again from comparing subsets of children who may have either disorder alone with those having their combination: for the present manual, children with RD only (N = 54), those having ADHD only (N = 102), and those having both disorders (RD + ADHD; N = 23). As before, the omnibus ANOVAs were all significant (all p's < .001). The results are shown in Figure 7.7. Pairwise contrasts again revealed unique patterns of EF deficits for the two disorders. For the Self-Management to Time and Self-Organization/Problem Solving subscales, the groups differed significantly from each other in a sequential order of severity: RD + ADHD > ADHD only > RD only > controls. In these domains, both disorders have some adverse effects, though clearly ADHD has greater effects than RD. And those effects appear to be additive, suggesting some unique influence of each disorder on these domains. But for the remaining scales (Self-Restraint, Self-Motivation, and Self-Regulation of Emotion), only the two ADHD groups differed from the controls and the RD-only groups; the latter two groups were not different in these domains. Again, we see here that ADHD has its usual pervasive impact on all EF domains, whereas RD has a unique impact only on Self-Management to Time and Self-Organization/Problem Solving domains.

Spelling Disorders

Spelling disorders (SpD) have been far less studied in children and are typically collapsed in children having RD because of a strong relationship between them and because both often share a common association with language problems more generally and phonological awareness and decoding specifically (Lewis, Freebairn, & Taylor, 2002; Warnke, 1999). Again, following the same logic as for SLD and RD, the importance of language to the development of verbal working memory and

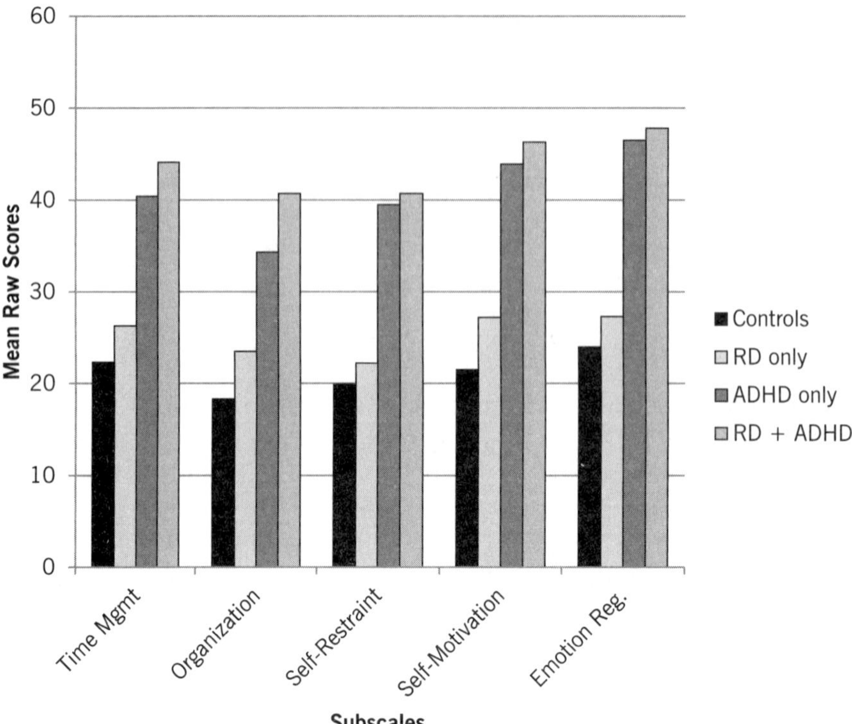

FIGURE 7.7. Raw scores for the BDEFS-CA subscales for children who had received a professional diagnosis of reading disorder (RD) alone, those with ADHD alone, those with both disorders (RD + ADHD) and the remainder of the sample (controls). Time Mgmt, Self-Management to Time subscale; Organization, Self-Organization/Problem Solving subscale; Emotion Reg., Self-Regulation of Emotion subscale.

other EF components would suggest that children with SpD would be likely to have some deficits in EF. But there is little or no research on the EF deficits associated with SpD independently of ADHD, whether using psychometric tests or parent ratings of EF. To do so here, children in the original sample having SpD ($N = 45$) were compared with those without SpD ($N = 1,877$). As expected, the groups differed significantly on all 10 scores from the BDEFS-CA (all p's < .001). Yet, once again, the specter of comorbidity with ADHD and SpD is problematic. It has been suggested that 15–25% of children with ADHD may have an SpD (Barkley, 2006), though the inverse association has been little studied. Even so, given the high comorbidity of SpD with RD and of both with SLD and the fact that children with RD and SLD have elevated rates of ADHD, it is conceivable that ADHD is overrepresented in children with SpD. Following the same procedure as with the other learning disabilities, the analyses here were repeated, with those children having ADHD removed (reduced N's = 33 and 1,764, respectively). All comparisons remained significant (all p's < .003 except Self-Restraint, which was $p < .02$); those results appear in Table 7.12.

More interesting and important for determining validity, again, is the pattern of EF deficits among children with SpD only ($N = 33$) in comparison with children with ADHD only (N = 113) or those having both disorders (N = 12; SpD + ADHD) relative to the control-group children (N = 1,764). These groups were compared on all five BDEFS-CA subscales, and the omnibus ANOVAs were all significant (all p's < .001). The results are shown in Figure 7.8. The pairwise comparisons for the Self-Management to Time, Self-Organization/Problem Solving, and Self-Motivation scales showed the same pattern; all the groups differed from each other by order of severity: SpD + ADHD > ADHD only > SpD only > controls. These results imply that both ADHD and SpD contribute to EF deficits but that ADHD does so more than SpD. The fact that the comorbid group is the most abnormal also implies that SpD may make some unique contributions to EF apart from ADHD and that the effects of both disorders are additive when comorbid. The pattern for the Self-Restraint scale shows that it is associated only with ADHD in that both ADHD groups differed significantly from the SpD-only and control groups, who did not differ. Yet even here the children in the comorbid condition had significantly greater EF deficits than did the ADHD-only group. An even different pattern emerged for the Self-Regulation of Emotion scale. Here, both ADHD groups had higher scores than either the SpD-only or control group, and the two ADHD groups did not differ in severity of EF deficits. But the SpD-only group also had higher scores on this scale than did the control group, even if this difference was substantially smaller than that associated with the ADHD groups. Again, SpD alone may have some impact on this dimension of EF even if ADHD is by far a worse disorder in its impact on EF. Once more, such differential patterns are both informative about the nature of the relationship between SpD and EF deficits and also important for establishing the validity of the BDEFS-CA.

TABLE 7.12. BDEFS-CA Long and Short Form Scores for Children with and without a Professional Diagnosis of SpD (without ADHD)

	No SpD (no ADHD) (N = 1,764)		SpD (no ADHD) (N = 33)			
Subscale	Mean	*SD*	Mean	*SD*	*F*	*p*
Self-Management to Time	22.3	7.5	27.2	6.6	14.00	< .001
Self-Organization	18.4	5.7	23.1	6.7	21.85	< .001
Self-Restraint	19.9	6.7	22.7	6.1	5.53	.019
Self-Motivation	21.6	7.8	28.1	7.9	23.02	< .001
Self-Reg. of Emotion	24.0	8.8	28.6	8.3	9.05	.003
Total EF Summary Score	106.3	30.9	129.9	26.8	18.97	< .001
ADHD-EF Index	14.5	4.2	18.0	4.0	23.83	< .001
EF Symptom Count	6.1	10.3	12.5	11.4	12.63	< .001
EF Summary Score—Short Form	31.2	9.1	38.0	7.3	18.22	< .001
EF Symptom Count—Short Form	2.0	3.2	3.7	3.2	9.28	< .001

Note. SpD, spelling disorder; F, results for the F-test; p, probability value for the F-test if ≤ .05; Self-Organization, Self-Organization/Problem Solving subscale; Self-Reg. of Emotion, Self-Regulation of Emotion subscale.

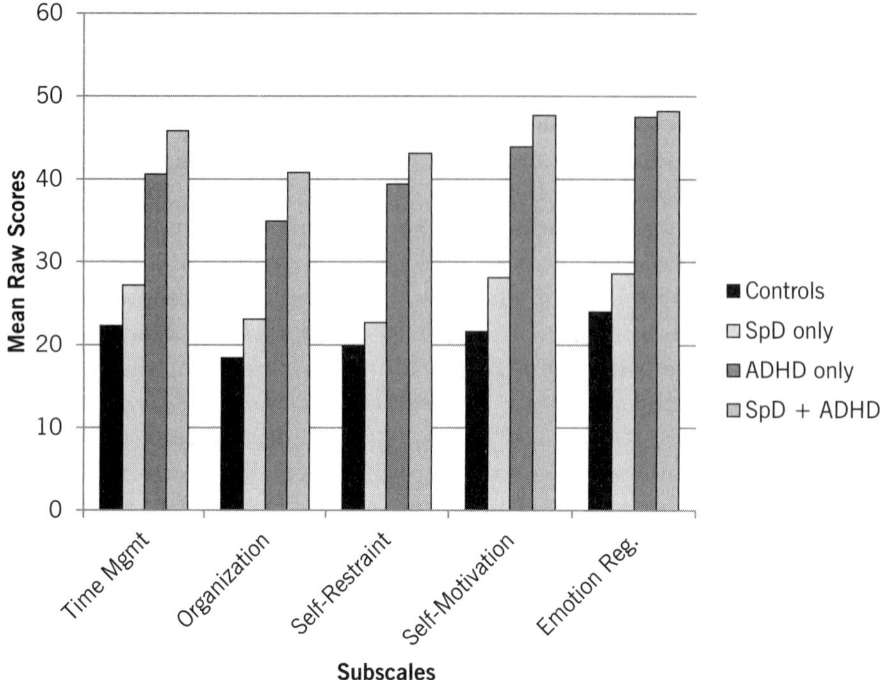

FIGURE 7.8. Raw scores for the BDEFS-CA subscales for children who had received a professional diagnosis of spelling disorder (SpD) alone, those with ADHD alone, those with both disorders (SpD + ADHD) and the remainder of the sample (controls). Time Mgmt, Self-Management to Time subscale; Organization, Self-Organization/Problem Solving subscale; Emotion Reg., Self-Regulation of Emotion subscale.

Math Disorders

Studies suggest that approximately 3–8% of school-age children have math disorders (MD) (Swanson & Jerman, 2006). Research comparing such children with typical children often finds them to be deficient on psychometric measures of both verbal and nonverbal (visual–spatial) working memory, as well as of nonexecutive abilities such as naming speed, processing speed, and long-term memory (Geary, Hoard, Byrd-Craven, Nugent, & Numtee, 2007; see meta-analysis by Swanson & Jerman, 2006). However, in comparison with children with RD, studies indicate that verbal and nonverbal working memory and processing speed are the main concomitants of MD. When controlling for other potential confounding variables (IQ, age, etc.), differences between these groups have been shown to be largely mediated by the deficits in both verbal and nonverbal working memory (Swanson & Jerman, 2006), two important components of EF. One would therefore expect children with a history of math disorders to demonstrate greater deficits on parental ratings of EF, such as on the BDEFS-CA, but to be substantially less impaired in this regard than children with ADHD. No prior research could be located that has made such comparisons on parent EF ratings.

Approximately 2% of the original sample had parental reports of a diagnosis of MD ($N = 44$). These children were compared with the remainder of the sample (N

= 1,878) on the BDEFS-CA scores. Consistent with the prior studies discussed, significant differences were evident on all scores (all *p*'s < .001). Once again, however, children with MD may also have ADHD and vice versa at higher rates than expected by chance; the overlap with ADHD might account for the group differences on EF measures. It has been estimated that 10–18% of children with ADHD may also have MD (Capano, Minden, Chen, Schachar, & Ickowicz, 2008; Del'Homme et al., 2007). Children with ADHD were removed from the groups and the comparisons made again between the MD-only children (*N* = 29) and the remainder (N = 1,768). All comparisons remained significant and are shown in Table 7.13.

As was done previously, additional analyses were then conducted to evaluate the pattern of EF deficits in MD relative to ADHD. Comparisons were made among those children with MD only (*N* = 29), those with ADHD only (*N* = 110), and those having the comorbid condition (MD + ADHD; *N* = 15); these three groups were also compared with the control group (*N* = 1,768). The omnibus ANOVAs for the five BDEFS-CA subscales were all significant (all *p*'s < .001). The results are shown in Figure 7.9. The pairwise comparisons once again revealed a different pattern of results for MD in contrast to ADHD. On all five scales, the two groups with ADHD scored significantly worse than those with MD only and the controls, with the two ADHD groups not differing in their severity of deficits. And for the Self-Restraint subscale, the MD-only and control groups did not differ from each other. But on the other four scales, MD only was associated with higher EF deficits compared with controls, even if these deficits were not of the severity associated with ADHD. Those EF deficits did not contribute in any additive way when the two disorders were comorbid. MD, like all of the learning disorders discussed previously, may have some relationship to ADHD symptom severity even in those cases that do not meet the research diagnostic criteria imposed here to define cases of ADHD. This

TABLE 7.13. BDEFS-CA Long and Short Form Scores for Children with and without a Professional Diagnosis of MD (without ADHD)

	No MD (no ADHD) (*N* = 1,768)		MD (no ADHD) (*N* = 29)			
Subscale	Mean	*SD*	Mean	*SD*	*F*	*p*
Self-Management to Time	22.3	7.4	28.7	7.3	21.06	< .001
Self-Organization	18.4	5.6	26.5	8.1	57.62	< .001
Self-Restraint	19.9	6.7	22.5	6.9	4.13	.042
Self-Motivation	21.6	7.7	29.9	7.8	32.50	< .001
Self-Reg. of Emotion	24.0	8.8	28.5	9.0	7.52	.006
Total EF Summary Score	106.2	30.8	136.1	31.2	26.81	< .001
ADHD-EF Index	14.4	4.1	19.3	4.6	39.30	< .001
EF Symptom Count	6.0	10.2	16.4	13.2	28.83	< .001
EF Summary Score—Short Form	31.2	9.0	39.7	8.3	25.43	< .001
EF Symptom Count—Short Form	2.0	3.2	4.9	3.5	24.16	< .001

Note. MD, math disorder; *F*, results for the *F*-test; *p*, probability value for the *F*-test if ≤ .05; Self-Organization, Self-Organization/Problem Solving subscale; Self-Reg. of Emotion, Self-Regulation of Emotion subscale.

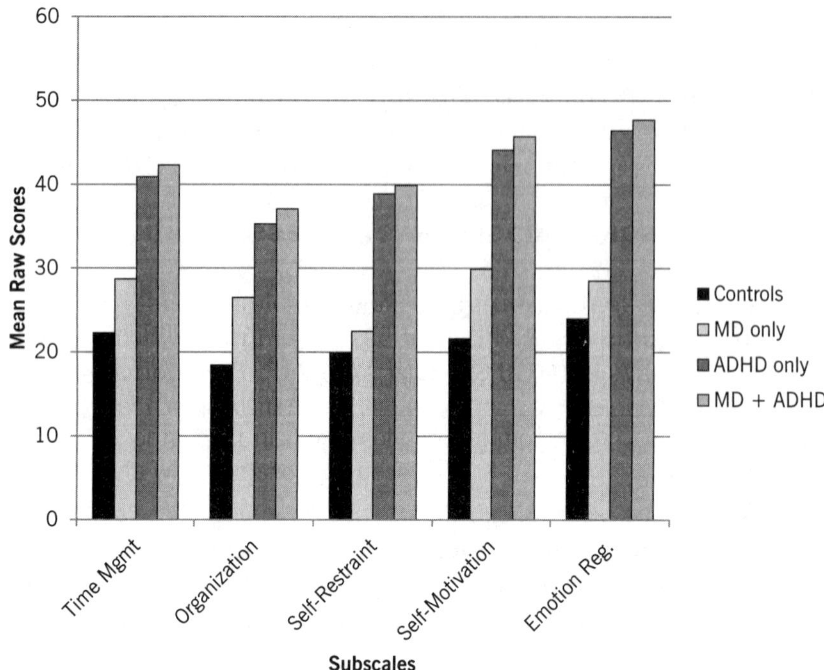

FIGURE 7.9. Raw scores for the BDEFS-CA subscales for children who had received a professional diagnosis of math disorders (MD) alone, those with ADHD alone, those with both disorders (MD + ADHD) and the remainder of the sample (controls). Time Mgmt, Self-Management to Time subscale; Organization, Self-Organization/Problem Solving subscale; Emotion Reg., Self-Regulation of Emotion subscale.

might result in MD-only cases differing in their levels of EF deficits to a small but significant degree from the control group, while being much less affected in their EF deficits than is the case for fully diagnosed cases of ADHD. This would account for the fact that MD added no additional EF deficits when comorbid with ADHD beyond those seen in ADHD alone.

Another case in which differential patterns of EF deficits may be of interest concerns the differences between children who have MD only, those who have RD only, and those with both conditions. Typically, these two disorders can coexist at higher rates than expected from their base rates, but they can also occur independently (Swanson & Jerman, 2006). But as discussed earlier, they may have some distinct associations with different measures of EF, at least as assessed by psychometric tests. To explore this possibility, children with MD only ($N = 6$) were compared with those with RD only ($N = 31$), those with both disorders (MD + RD; $N = 23$), and the remainder of the sample (control; $N = 1,737$). Any children with ADHD were removed from these comparisons given the overrepresentation of that disorder in these conditions (Del'Homme et al., 2007) and in case of any differential association of ADHD with these other disorders. The small number of children with MD limits the power of the comparison of that group with the others, and so this analysis is more exploratory than definitive. All of the omnibus ANOVAs were significant (all p's < .001). The findings are shown in Figure 7.10.

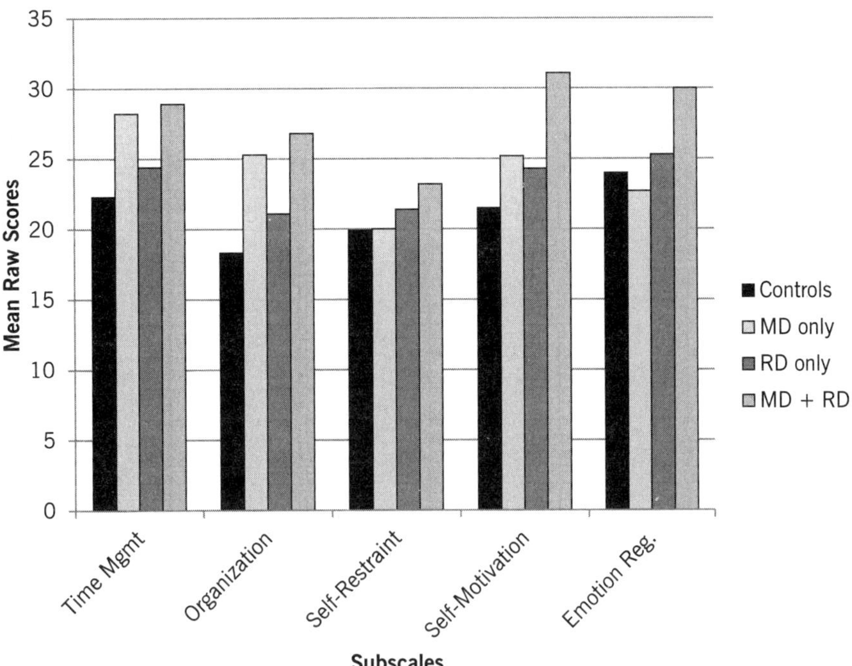

FIGURE 7.10. Raw scores for the BDEFS-CA subscales for children who had received a professional diagnosis of MD alone, RD only, those with both disorders (MD + RD), and the remainder of the sample (controls). All children with ADHD were removed from these groups. Time Mgmt, Self-Management to Time subscale; Organization, Self-Organization/Problem Solving subscale; Emotion Reg., Self-Regulation of Emotion subscale.

The pairwise comparisons showed that only the two groups having MD had significant difficulties on the Self-Management to Time subscale and the Self-Organization/Problem Solving scale compared with the other two groups, whereas those with RD only did not differ from the controls. And only the comorbid MD + RD group had any significant problems with Self-Motivation. In contrast, only the groups with RD were significantly different on the Self-Regulation of Emotion scale from both the MD-only and control groups, who did not differ. This is a double dissociation in which one disorder has a distinctly different pattern of EF deficits than the other disorder; effects were not additive on most scales when the comorbid condition exists, with the exception of the Self-Motivation scale, on which only that comorbid condition yielded a significant impact. Given the small sample sizes and limited power for the groups, the results were reanalyzed, treating MD and RD as separate factors in a two-way ANOVA. The results essentially corroborated the preceding interpretations. There was a significant main effect ($p < .001$) for MD only on the Self-Management to Time and Self-Organization/Problem Solving scales. Neither disorder affected the Self-Restraint scale, which, as shown earlier, is primarily associated with ADHD. Again, as previously, only RD was associated with difficulties on the Self-Regulation of Emotion subscale. On the Self-Motivation scale, both disorders produced a significant main effect yet did not interact significantly with each other. In sum, the double dissociation was replicated, with MD having an adverse effect on the time management and self-organization domains, whereas RD had an adverse effect on emotional self-regulation; both disorders adversely influenced self-motivation. As shown, such findings are scientifically informative in their own right while also providing even more evidence for the criterion validity of the BDEFS-CA.

Writing Disorders

Following the same reasoning as previously for the other learning disabilities, writing disorders (WD) would likewise be expected to be associated with some deficits in EF given the linkage of language development to EF and to WD. Moreover, disorders of the prefrontal lobe, or executive brain, may result in WD, or executive agraphia, given the need for planning, problem solving, and verbal working memory in writing apart from the motor requirements of the act of writing itself (Ardila & Surloff, 2006). For this reason, children with a professional diagnosis of WD (N = 43) were compared with the remainder of the original sample (N = 1,879) on all BDEFS-CA scores. As might be expected, all comparisons were significant (all p's < .001). But, as with the other learning and language disorders, children with WD are at elevated risk for ADHD. Certainly children with ADHD have a significant rate of comorbid WD or, at the very least, difficulties with writing, even if they do not rise to the level of a WD (Barkley, 2006; Re, Pedron, & Cornoldi, 2007). For instance, Del'Homme and colleagues (2007) found that children with ADHD had WD in 16–24% of their cases, which is similar to reports from other studies (Barkley, 2006). So the group comparisons were repeated with the ADHD cases once again removed from both groups. All comparisons remained significant (all p's < .001). The results are shown in Table 7.14.

TABLE 7.14. BDEFS-CA Long and Short Form Scores for Children with and without a Professional Diagnosis of WD (without ADHD)

	No WD (no ADHD) (N = 1,769)		WD (no ADHD) (N = 28)			
Subscale	Mean	*SD*	Mean	*SD*	F	p
Self-Management to Time	22.3	7.5	28.0	6.7	16.08	< .001
Self-Organization	18.4	5.6	27.1	9.6	65.47	< .001
Self-Restraint	19.9	6.7	24.3	6.9	11.78	< .001
Self-Motivation	21.6	7.7	30.1	8.5	33.00	< .001
Self-Reg. of Emotion	24.0	8.8	29.9	8.5	12.47	< .001
Total EF Summary Score	106.2	30.8	139.5	30.4	32.22	< .001
ADHD-EF Index	14.4	4.1	19.7	4.9	44.73	< .001
EF Symptom Count	6.0	10.2	17.9	13.4	37.11	< .001
EF Summary Score—Short Form	31.2	9.0	40.2	8.4	27.75	< .001
EF Symptom Count—Short Form	2.0	3.2	4.9	3.7	23.83	< .001

Note. WD, writing disorder; F, results for the F-test; p, probability value for the F-test if ≤ .05; Self-Organization, Self-Organization/Problem Solving subscale; Self-Reg. of Emotion, Self-Regulation of Emotion subscale.

Following the same logic used before, it is even more informative to examine the impact of WD alone (*N* = 28), that of ADHD alone (*N* = 110) and the combination of the two disorders (WD + ADHD, *N* = 15) in comparison with the control group (*N* = 1,769). These comparisons were made on the five BDEFS-CA subscales and, as before, all omnibus ANOVAs were significant (at $p < .001$). The results are shown in Figure 7.11. Pairwise comparisons showed that the pattern on four of the five scales was identical: the two ADHD groups had significantly higher scores than the WD-only and control groups, but the two ADHD groups did not differ from each other. Once more, it is largely ADHD that is driving the deficits in EF in daily life. Even so, the WD-only group did have significantly higher scores than the controls, even though those scores were considerably below those for the two ADHD groups. Again, the effect of the two disorders coexisting did not yield any additive effects beyond those associated with ADHD alone. The exception to this pattern occurred on the Self-Regulation of Emotion subscale, on whcih all groups differed from each other, as follows: the ADHD-only group > WD + ADHD > WD only > controls. Here it is ADHD alone that is the most impairing, whereas the presence of a WD with ADHD seems to protect somewhat against these effects of ADHD. The effect here is not a direct one of additivity of the two disorders. Each disorder has its own effect on emotional self-regulation, but ADHD alone is clearly the most influential. As noted earlier, such evidence of distinctive patterns for different dis-

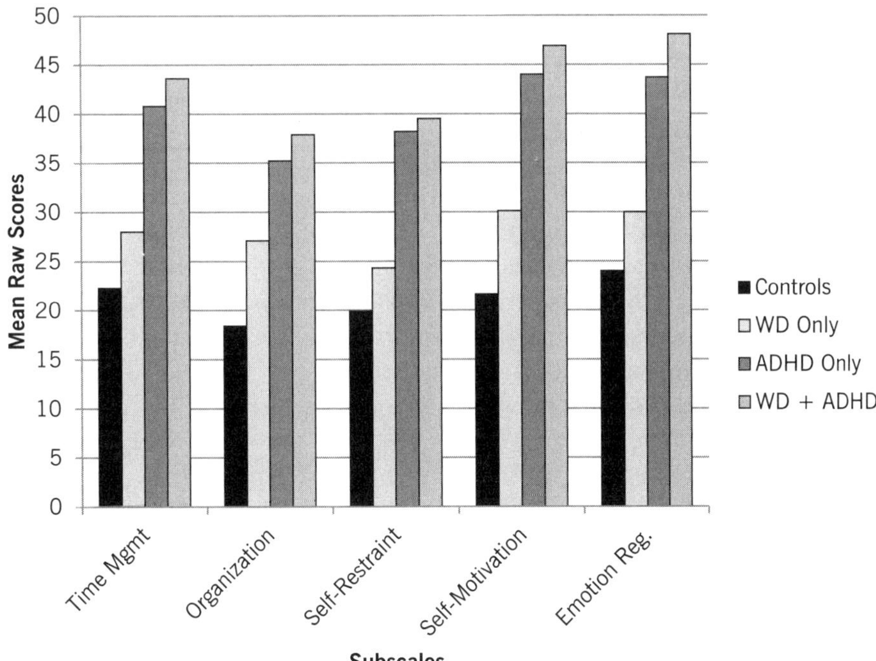

FIGURE 7.11. Raw scores for the BDEFS-CA subscales for children who had received a professional diagnosis of writing disorders (WD) alone, ADHD alone, those with both disorders (WD + ADHD), and the remainder of the sample (controls). Time Mgmt, Self-Management to Time subscale; Organization, Self-Organization/Problem Solving subscale; Emotion Reg., Self-Regulation of Emotion subscale.

orders and their coexistence provides considerable evidence for the validity of the BDEFS-CA apart from its scientific and clinical importance.

Psychiatric Disorders

Anxiety Disorders

Symptoms of anxiety or fears are commonplace in childhood. Rates of actual anxiety disorders in childhood vary widely across studies, from 2.6 to 41.2% (Cartwright-Hatton, McNicol, & Doubleday, 2006) and are clearly related to diagnostic criteria and ascertainment methods. But the prevalence of anxiety disorders during any 3- to 6-month period may be closer to 2–11% in childhood (Costello et al., 1996; Last, Perrin, Hersen, & Kazdin, 1996) and 8–19% in mid-adolescence (Essau, Conradt, & Petermann, 2000; Kashani & Orvaschel, 1988). There is a high rate of remission of anxiety disorders over a 3- to 4-year period in childhood (82%) and a small (8%) chance of relapse back to the original anxiety disorder. But some additional risk remains for the development of new psychiatric disorders (30%) (Last et al., 1996). Depression is the most common comorbidity (approximately 28%) with anxiety disorders by adolescence, but ADHD also exists in a significant minority of cases (Essau et al., 2000). There is little evidence that EF deficits exist in children with anxiety disorders, especially in comparison with other disorders, such as ADHD, in which significant difficulties may exist, as noted previously (Gunther, Holtkamp, Jolles, Herpertz-Dahlmann, & Konrad, 2004). But some studies have found patients with various anxiety disorders to perform poorly on EF tests of planning and problem solving and also on non-EF tests of episodic memory (Airaksinen, Larsson, & Forsell, 2005; Toren et al., 2000). Some evidence also suggests an adverse effect of anxiety disorders on verbal learning and memory (Toren et al., 2000). In contrast, children with anxiety disorders are unlikely to have deficits in response inhibition, a deficit most often associated with ADHD (Korenblum, Chen, Manassis, & Schachar, 2007; Oosterlaan, Logan, & Sergeant, 1998; Pliszka, 2009; Shatz & Rostain, 2006). It is therefore uncertain whether anxiety disorders are associated with EF deficits in daily life activities as assessed through parent ratings. Some research with children with Williams syndrome suggests their level of anxiety may be linked to parent-reported EF deficits in daily life activities (Woodruff-Borden, Kistler, Henderson, Crawford, & Mervis, 2010).

In the present sample, 56 children (2.9%) were reported by parents to have received professional diagnoses of anxiety disorders. This percentage is relatively low compared with the actual prevalence of the disorder in this age range and may have to do with the underdetection and hence underdiagnosis of such disorders by professionals. Or perhaps it is owing to the low agreement of parent- and child-reports of a child's anxiety and the fact that clinicians are less likely to directly interview children about their anxieties (Pliszka, 2009). Children with and without anxiety disorder diagnoses were compared on all 10 of the BDEFS-CA scores. The differences were substantial and significant in all comparisons (all p's < .001). Once again, however, ADHD can be a common comorbidity in children with anxiety disorders, being present in 17–35% of those children under 12 and at least 9% of adolescents (Pliszka, 2009; Shatz & Rostain, 2006; Tannock, 2009). The reverse is also the case, with 20–50% of children with ADHD having comorbid anxiety disorders (Pliszka, 2009; Shatz & Rostain, 2006; Tannock, 2009). The presence of ADHD often increases the risk for school failure and for additional mental health intervention than is the case in anxiety disorders alone (Hammerness et al., 2010) and may exacerbate the degree of anxiety in such comorbid cases even more so than comorbidity with ASD and chronic TD (Guttmann-Steinmetz, Gadow, De Vincent, & Crowell, 2010). Yet the presence of anxiety in cases of ADHD may reduce their inhibitory (Pliszka, 2009; Tannock, 2009) or attention (Vloet, Konrad, Herpertz-Dahlmann, Polier, & Gunther, 2010) problems. Given the substantial impact of ADHD on parent ratings of EF deficits as reported earlier, it was important to remove this subset of cases having ADHD from the sample and then to reanalyze the differences between children with and without diagnoses of anxiety disorders. Thirty-four children had anxiety disorders but did not meet research criteria for ADHD. They were compared with the remainder of the sample (N = 1,763) after children with ADHD were removed from both groups. The comparisons of these two groups are shown in Table 7.15. All remained significant, although the magnitude of the differences was now substantially reduced by removal of the ADHD cases, as would be expected. This makes it clear that anxiety disorders can interfere with EF in daily life activities whether or not they appear on psychometric tests of EF. This was also found to be the case in a study of children with Williams syndrome in which anxiety was associated with greater difficulties on the Behavioral Regulation scale of the BRIEF, perhaps owing to difficulties with emotional impulsiveness and poor emotional self-control (Woodruff-Borden et al., 2010).

Once again, however, the pattern that may exist among children with anxiety disorders alone (N = 34), those with ADHD alone (N = 103), and those with both

TABLE 7.15. BDEFS-CA Long and Short Form Scores for Children with and without a Professional Diagnosis of Anxiety Disorder (without ADHD)

	No anxiety disorder (no ADHD) (N = 1,763)		Anxiety disorder (no ADHD) (N = 34)			
Subscale	Mean	*SD*	Mean	*SD*	*F*	*p*
Self-Management to Time	22.3	7.5	25.8	6.4	6.91	.009
Self-Organization	18.4	5.7	21.6	8.2	10.23	.001
Self-Restraint	19.9	6.7	22.4	6.7	4.56	.033
Self-Motivation	21.6	7.8	26.1	9.5	11.18	.001
Self-Reg. of Emotion	23.9	8.7	31.5	10.0	24.91	< .001
Total EF Summary Score	106.3	30.8	127.5	33.8	15.67	< .001
ADHD-EF Index	14.5	4.1	17.2	5.2	14.60	< .001
EF Symptom Count	6.1	10.3	12.5	12.3	13.08	< .001
EF Summary Score—Short Form	31.2	9.0	36.4	9.7	10.71	.001
EF Symptom Count—Short Form	2.0	3.2	3.5	3.7	8.05	.005

Note. F = results for the F-test; p = probability value for the F-test if ≤ .05; Self-Organization, Self-Organization/Problem Solving subscale; Self-Reg. of Emotion, Self-Regulation of Emotion subscale.

disorders ($N = 22$) is important to examine for any evidence of a unique profile of EF deficits associated with each disorder and their co-occurrence. Again, the power of such comparisons may be limited given the small sample of cases having both disorders, but robust differences may still be evident. As with the other disorders, the five subscales of the BDEFS-CA were compared among these three groups and against the remainder of the sample ($N = 1,763$). All omnibus ANOVAs were significant (all p's $< .001$). The findings are graphically illustrated in Figure 7.12. The pairwise comparisons among the groups revealed a relatively distinct pattern for each disorder relative to the other. In all five comparisons, the two ADHD groups scored significantly worse than the controls or those with anxiety disorder alone. For the Self-Management to Time and Self-Motivation subscales, the two ADHD groups did not differ from each other. But for the remaining three scales, those with comorbid disorders had higher scores than those with ADHD alone, yet even the latter group always scored significantly worse than the anxiety-only group. The anxiety-disorder-only group had higher scores than the control group on the Self-Management to Time, Self-Organization/Problem Solving, Self-Motivation, and Self-Regulation of Emotion subscales but not on the Self-Restraint subscale, again suggesting that scores on that scale are more likely to be specifically related to

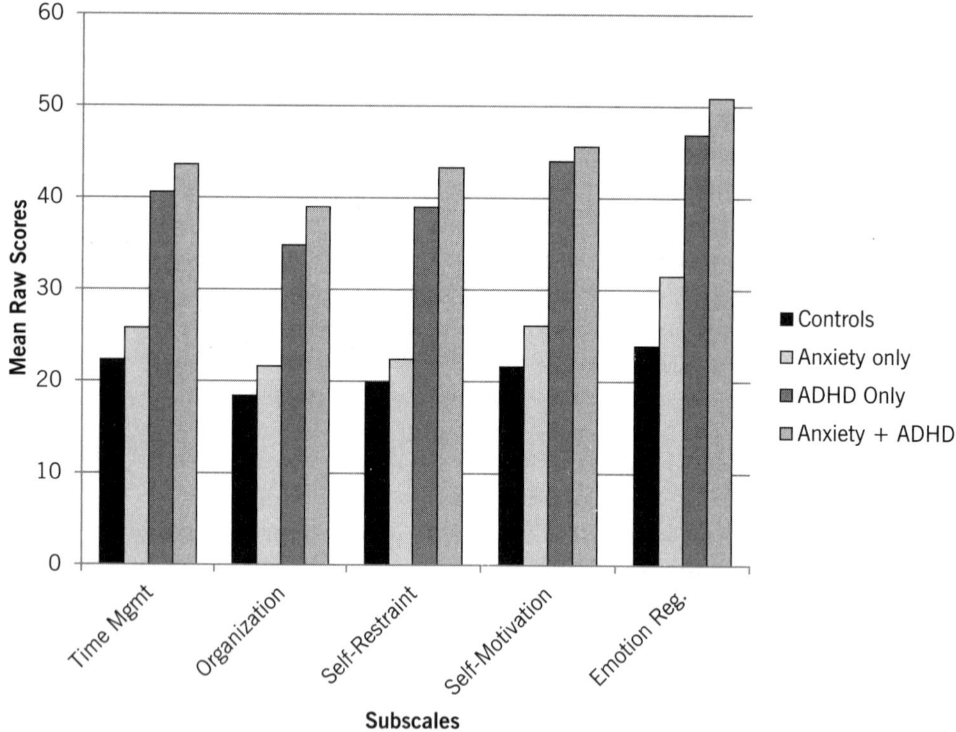

FIGURE 7.12. Raw scores for the BDEFS-CA subscales for children who had received a professional diagnosis of any anxiety disorders alone, ADHD alone, those with both disorders (anxiety + ADHD), and the remainder of the sample (controls). Time Mgmt, Self-Management to Time subscale; Organization, Self-Organization/Problem Solving subscale; Emotion Reg., Self-Regulation of Emotion subscale.

ADHD and not to anxiety disorders. This has certainly been the case when tests of inhibition have been used to compare these two disorders (Korenblum et al., 2007; Oosterlaan et al., 1998; Pliszka, 2009). For two of the scales (Self-Organization/Problem Solving and Self-Regulation of Emotion), the level of EF deficits increased significantly across the groups such that all groups differed from each other as follows and each disorder had an additive effect when comorbid: anxiety + ADHD > ADHD only > anxiety only > controls. In summary, ADHD has a substantially more negative impact on EF in daily life activities in children than do anxiety disorders, especially on scales pertaining to time management and self-restraint or inhibition. But anxiety disorders make their own contribution, even if a smaller one, to the three other parent-rated domains of EF.

Depression

The rate of depression in childhood ranges from 2 to 10% (Fleming, Offord, & Boyle, 1989; Kashani et al., 1983; Lefkowitz & Tesiny, 1985; Lewinsohn, Hops, Roberts, Seeley, & Andrews, 1993; Son & Kirchner, 2000) and is higher (5–8%) in adolescence (Son & Kirchner, 2000), with a lifetime prevalence rate by adolescence of 33% (Lewinsohn et al., 1993). Although depression may occur alone in children, it is typically associated with anxiety in 16–62% of all cases (Kendall, 1992), among other disorders. Limited evidence exists as to whether EF deficits are associated with depression in children, but what little does exist shows an adverse effect on EF tests (Jonsdottir et al., 2006) such as sequencing and problem solving (Emerson, Mollet, & Harrison, 2005), as well as a detrimental effect on verbal memory (Gunther et al., 2004). This is in contrast to anxiety disorders where no such deficit in memory seems to occur (Gunther et al., 2004). There is, consequently, some likelihood that children with depression are likely to do poorly on parent ratings of EF in daily life activities though this possibility does not seem to have been previously studied.

Parents reported professional diagnoses of depression for 32 children in this sample (1.6%). This rate is toward the lower end of the range found in epidemiological studies (see previous discussion). Again, as with anxiety disorders, this finding could result from low agreement between parents and children about a child's depressive symptoms or mood states, from limited efforts to detect depression in children by professionals, and from limitations in the DSM criteria for depression when applied to children (Pliszka, 2009). When these children were compared with the remainder of the sample on all BDEFS-CA scores, substantial and significant differences were evident in all comparisons (all p's < .001). Here again, there is a possibility of depression being contaminated with comorbid ADHD. As many as 20–50% of children with depression may have ADHD, and 20–30% or more of children with ADHD may have depression (Carlson & Meyer, 2009; Pliszka, 2009). When the ADHD cases ($N = 9$) were removed from the depressed group and the control group, all differences remained significant. Those analyses are shown in Table 7.16. Thus depression in children, even in the absence of comorbid ADHD, is associated with pervasive effects on EF in daily life. Of greater interest is whether this effect shows a unique pattern relative to children with ADHD only or to those with both disorders. To evaluate these patterns, children with depression only ($N = 23$) were compared with those with ADHD only ($N = 116$) and those with both

TABLE 7.16. BDEFS-CA Long and Short Form Scores for Children with and without a Professional Diagnosis of Depression (without ADHD)

	No depression (No ADHD) (*N* = 1,774)		Depression (No ADHD) (*N* = 23)			
Subscale	Mean	*SD*	Mean	*SD*	*F*	*p*
Self-Management to Time	22.3	7.4	29.6	7.1	21.39	< .001
Self-Organization	18.4	5.7	23.2	9.0	15.52	< .001
Self-Restraint	19.9	6.7	25.3	7.9	14.56	< .001
Self-Motivation	21.6	7.7	29.7	9.8	25.54	< .001
Self-Reg. of Emotion	23.9	8.7	34.5	9.8	33.29	< .001
Total EF Summary Score	106.2	30.7	142.3	36.7	31.15	< .001
ADHD-EF Index	14.5	4.1	19.0	5.0	27.51	< .001
EF Symptom Count	6.1	10.2	17.1	16.4	26.09	< .001
EF Summary Score—Short Form	31.2	9.0	41.5	9.8	29.71	< .001
EF Symptom Count—Short Form	2.0	3.1	5.2	4.8	22.95	< .001

Note. F = results for the *F*-test; *p* = probability value for the *F*-test if ≤ .05; Self-Organization, Self-Organization/Problem Solving subscale; Self-Reg. of Emotion, Self-Regulation of Emotion subscale.

disorders (*N* = 9), as well as with the remainder of the sample (*N* = 1,774) on the five BDEFS-CA subscales. These results can be seen in Figure 7.13. The power for the comorbid sample is quite low, however, and may obscure group differences that are less than large or robust. Even so, an interesting pattern of results emerged from the pairwise comparisons—one that was quite different from that seen for anxiety disorders. On all five scales, all groups were significantly different from each other. There was evidence of additivity between the two disorders on all scales, as shown in the following sequence of severity across groups: depression + ADHD > ADHD only > depression only > controls. It is clear from this pattern that ADHD alone is associated with greater deficits in EF than is depression alone across all of the subscales. But depression alone is associated with greater EF deficits than in the control group for all of the scales as well. And the comorbid group, small as it was, always had the greatest deficits in EF ratings on all scales, implying some additivity of their effects beyond that seen in either disorder alone.

Just as useful for substantiating the validity of the BDEFS-CA is an analysis of the pattern of EF deficits between cases with depression and those with anxiety disorder. Given that anxiety is often present in cases of depression and vice versa, it is useful to see what EF deficits are associated with each disorder alone and combined. Of course, the comorbidity of each with ADHD would need to be controlled (removed). Unfortunately, in this sample, just 5 children had comorbid depression and anxiety when cases of ADHD were removed from the sample. But 29 children had anxiety only and 18 depression only without a research diagnosis of ADHD. These cases were compared against each other and the remainder of the sample (*N* = 1,745) on the five BDEFS-CA subscales. All omnibus ANOVAs were significant at the $p < .001$ level. The results are shown in Figure 7.14. The sample sizes are admittedly small, and thus power to detect group differences is probably restricted

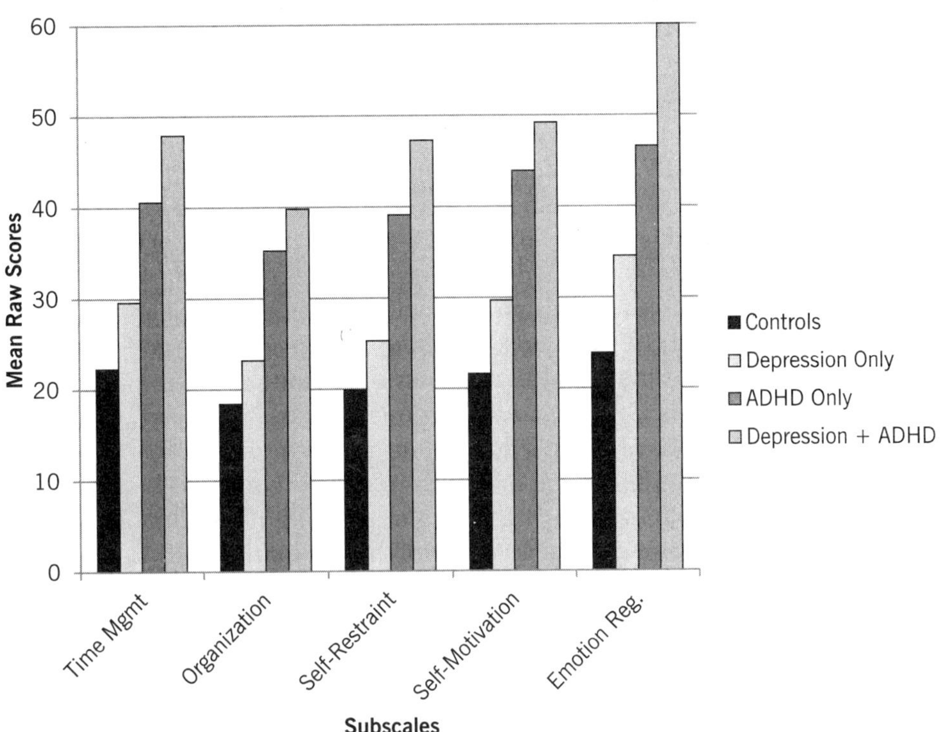

FIGURE 7.13. Raw scores for the BDEFS-CA subscales for children who had received a professional diagnosis of any depression disorders alone, ADHD alone, those with both disorders (depression + ADHD), and the remainder of the sample (controls). Time Mgmt, Self-Management to Time subscale; Organization, Self-Organization/Problem Solving subscale; Emotion Reg., Self-Regulation of Emotion subscale.

to large effect sizes. Nonetheless, some unique patterns emerged in the pairwise comparisons. Children with depression only had higher scores on all five subscales than did control-group children. Children with anxiety only, in contrast, were not different from the control group on three of the scales (Self-Management to Time, Self-Restraint, and Self-Motivation). But they did differ from the control group on the Self-Organization/Problem Solving and Self-Regulation of Emotion subscales. On these scales, they did not differ from those with depression only. These results suggest that depression has a pervasive adverse impact across all five domains of EF in daily life, whereas anxiety has a more selective adverse effect on organization and problem solving, as well as emotional self-regulation, but not on self-restraint (inhibition), self-motivation, or time management. Once more, these results and those for anxiety disorders are not only of scientific interest but also of considerable importance in validating the BDEFS-CA scores.

Bipolar Disorder

Just 14 of the children in the original sample carried a professional diagnosis of bipolar disorder (BPD) or manic–depression, according to parents. This rate is

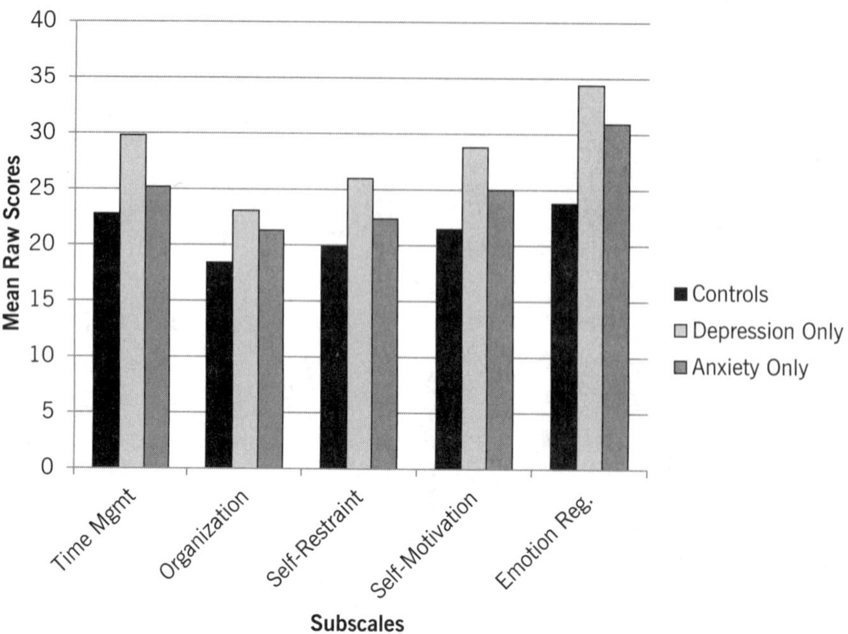

FIGURE 7.14. Raw scores for the BDEFS-CA subscales for children who had received a professional diagnosis of any depression disorders alone, any anxiety disorders alone, and the remainder of the sample (controls), with all cases of ADHD removed. Time Mgmt, Self-Management to Time subscale; Organization, Self-Organization/Problem Solving subscale; Emotion Reg., Self-Regulation of Emotion subscale.

well below that found in epidemiological studies, in which up to 6% of children may meet criteria for BPD, averaging about 1.8% (Youngstrom, Arnold, & Frazier, 2010). BPD is associated with significant difficulties across most domains of EF as assessed psychometrically (Walshaw, Alloy, & Sabb, 2010), but deficits may be especially prominent on measures of planning, set shifting, and interference control relative to ADHD. The results for these 14 children were compared with the rest of the sample. All of the comparisons were significant ($p < .001$), and substantial differences emerged. Indeed, the mean differences are among the largest for any disorder other than ADHD. Problematic in EF research on BPD and in these comparisons is the substantial overlap or comorbidity of BPD with ADHD, averaging 62% (Youngstrom et al., 2010). Consistent with these findings, 7 of the 14 children with BPD in this small sample also met the criteria for a research diagnosis of ADHD. As with the other disorders discussed, the cases of comorbid ADHD were removed, and the comparisons were redone. These results are shown in Table 7.17. Despite the exceptionally small group with BPD only ($N = 7$), all results remained significant and were still substantial in magnitude.

Just as with the other disorders, children with BPD only were compared with the group with ADHD only and with the group having both BPD and ADHD ($N = 7$) on the BDEFS-CA five subscales. All omnibus ANOVAs were significant at $p < .001$. Those findings are portrayed in Figure 7.15. The pairwise contrasts were most informative in showing that both ADHD groups scored worse than the BPD-

TABLE 7.17. BDEFS-CA Long and Short Form Scores for Children with and without a Professional Diagnosis of BPD (without ADHD)

	No BPD (no ADHD) (*N* = 1,790)		BPD (no ADHD) (*N* = 7)			
Subscale	Mean	*SD*	Mean	*SD*	*F*	*p*
Self-Management to Time	22.3	7.5	31.5	5.7	10.52	.001
Self-Organization	18.5	5.8	25.4	6.7	10.08	.002
Self-Restraint	19.9	6.7	32.3	8.4	23.67	< .001
Self-Motivation	21.7	7.8	31.7	8.7	11.54	.001
Self-Reg. of Emotion	24.0	8.7	42.6	10.6	31.42	< .001
Total EF Summary Score	106.5	30.8	163.6	32.6	23.88	< .001
ADHD-EF Index	14.5	4.2	21.0	3.5	16.95	< .001
EF Symptom Count	6.1	10.2	26.1	15.9	23.39	< .001
EF Summary Score—Short Form	31.3	9.0	45.8	8.1	18.11	< .001
EF Symptom Count—Short Form	2.0	3.2	6.8	4.6	16.23	< .001

Note. BPD, bipolar disorder; *F* = results for the *F*-test; *p* = probability value for the *F*-test if ≤ .05; Self-Organization, Self-Organization/Problem Solving subscale; Self-Reg. of Emotion, Self-Regulation of Emotion subscale.

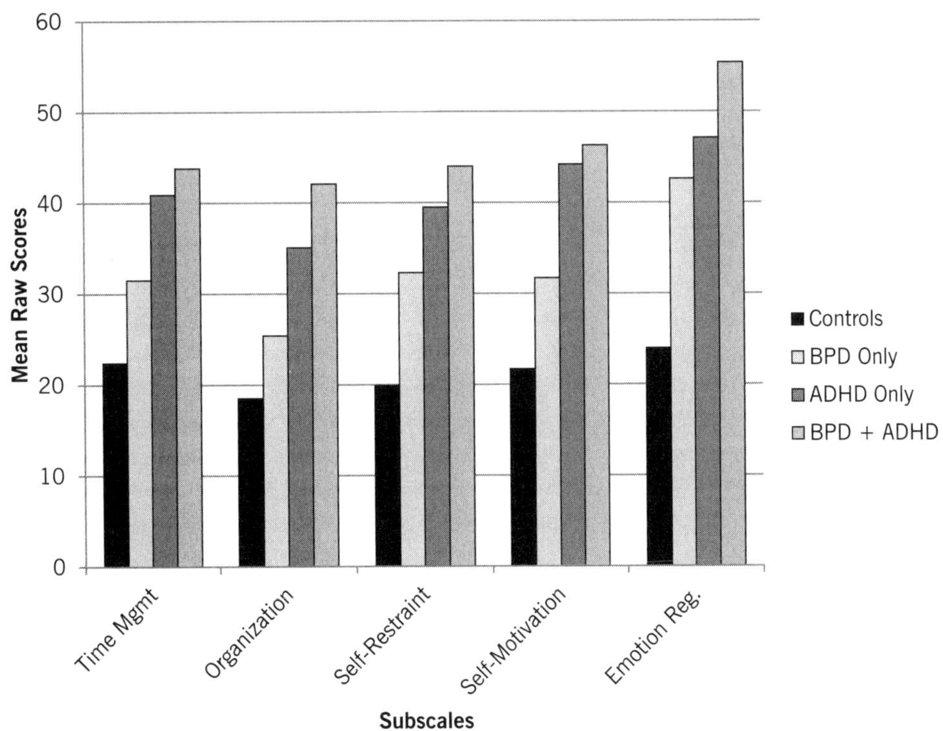

FIGURE 7.15. Raw scores for the BDEFS-CA subscales for children who had received a professional diagnosis of bipolar disorder or manic-depression (BPD) alone, to those with ADHD alone, those having both disorders (BPD + ADHD), and the remainder of the sample (controls). Time Mgmt, Self-Management to Time subscale; Organization, Self-Organization/Problem Solving subscale; Emotion Reg., Self-Regulation of Emotion subscale.

only group on three of the subscales: Self-Management to Time, Self-Restraint, and Self-Motivation. The BPD-only cases also differed from the control group on these three scales but had significantly lower scores than did either of the two groups with ADHD, which did not differ from each other. This finding suggests that although BPD may have some adverse effects on these domains, ADHD has significantly worse effects, and there is no additive effect of the comorbid condition. However, on the Self-Organization/Problem Solving subscale, all four groups differed significantly and showed evidence of additive effects: BPD + ADHD > ADHD only > BPD only > controls. On the Self-Regulation of Emotion subscale, the comorbid group was significantly worse than all other groups. The ADHD-only and BPD-only groups did not differ from each other, but both of these groups differed from the control group on this subscale. Given the nature of this scale and the fact that both ADHD and BPD are theorized to involve difficulties with emotion regulation, those with both disorders would be expected to be the most severely affected group.

Because of these small sample sizes in such pairwise comparisons, another way to analyze these results to find the distinct effect of BPD on EF is to compare those children with BPD and controls while statistically removing (covarying) the severity of ADHD symptoms. When this is done, the effect of BPD on Self-Management to Time and Self-Motivation is not significant, implying that BPD has no impact on these EF domains in the absence of ADHD symptoms. In contrast, the adverse impact of BPD on the remaining scales remained significant even after covarying ADHD severity. This implies that BPD has independent adverse effects on Self-Organization/Problem Solving, Self-Restraint, and Self-Regulation of Emotions independent of ADHD.

Oppositional Defiant Disorder

Prevalence estimates for oppositional defiant disorder (ODD) in the child population range from 2 to 16% (American Psychiatric Association, 2000). But more precise estimates place the number at 4–6% for children and 1–3% for adolescents (Barkley, 1997b). ODD alone has not been well studied for its association with deficits in EF, either on tests or on parent ratings. The disorder is often highly comorbid with ADHD as it is present in 40–60% of all ODD cases. The inverse is also the case: 40–84% or more of children with ADHD also have ODD (Barkley, 2006; Newcorn, Halperin, & Miller, 2009; Pliszka, 2009). Indeed, some have recently argued that ADHD may cause ODD, or at least contribute substantially to that component of the ODD associated with emotional impulsiveness and poor emotional self-regulation (Barkley, 2010). The social conflict component of ODD likely arises from disrupted parenting (Barkley, 2010). Most deficits in EF that have been shown to exist in such comorbid cases are typically ascribed to the existence of ADHD rather than to the ODD (Oosterlaan, Scheres, & Sergeant, 2005). The reason is often that the results for comorbid cases typically are not different from those having ADHD alone (Barnett, Maruff, & Vance, 2009; Qian, Shuai, Cao, Chan, & Wang, 2010). However, some research suggests that in adolescents, comorbidity with ODD (or conduct disorder) may create an even worse pattern on EF testing than is seen in ADHD alone (Hummer et al., 2011). It is therefore unclear from the results of psychometric EF tests whether ODD would be associated with deficits in parent ratings of EF in daily life, especially in the absence of ADHD. One recent study did use the BRIEF scale with Chinese children having ADHD only and having ADHD and ODD and reported more severe ratings for the comorbid group than was seen in the ADHD-only group, which also had higher scores than the control group. Such findings would imply that the greatest deficits in EF on the BDEFS-CA would be in the comorbid group given the high correlation of BDEFS-CA scores with those from the BRIEF for children (see the earlier discussion).

Just 28 children (1.4%) in the sample had received professional diagnoses of ODD, according to parental reports. As noted in Chapter 4, this low rate of diagnosis relative to rates of prevalence of ODD in the population is not uncommon given the reluctance of nonpsychiatric physicians to employ this diagnosis with children, at least in my experience. When the children with ODD were compared with those without ODD on the 10 BDEFS-CA scores, all comparisons were significant at $p < .001$. But the high comorbidity of ADHD with ODD may be contributing to this finding. Seventeen of the children with ODD also had ADHD (61%), consistent with the findings here of the high degree of comorbidity among the two disorders. So the comparisons were redone removing the ADHD cases; this left just 11 children having ODD alone. Even so, all results remained significant at $p < .001$. Those results appear in Table 7.18.

As with all of the other disorders discussed herein, it is useful to explore the pattern of findings among children having ODD only (N = 11), those with ADHD only (N = 108), and those having both disorders (N = 17) and the remainder of the sample (N = 1,786). The results of these comparisons are illustrated in Figure 7.16. The pairwise comparisons showed that ADHD only was always associated with higher scores than ODD only and controls. But the ODD-only group had higher scores

TABLE 7.18. BDEFS-CA Long and Short Form Scores for Children with and without a Professional Diagnosis of ODD (without ADHD)

	No ODD (no ADHD) (N = 1,786)		ODD (no ADHD) (N = 11)			
Subscale	Mean	*SD*	Mean	*SD*	*F*	*p*
Self-Management to Time	22.3	7.5	31.1	5.5	14.91	< .001
Self-Organization	18.5	5.8	25.9	6.0	18.24	< .001
Self-Restraint	19.9	6.7	31.2	5.8	31.00	< .001
Self-Motivation	21.7	7.8	30.4	8.0	13.61	< .001
Self-Reg. of Emotion	24.0	8.7	37.7	9.6	26.91	< .001
Total EF Summary Score	106.4	30.8	156.3	23.3	28.65	< .001
ADHD-EF Index	14.5	4.2	21.0	2.9	26.84	< .001
EF Symptom Count	6.1	10.2	22.4	13.9	27.30	< .001
EF Summary Score—Short Form	31.2	9.0	45.5	7.8	27.44	< .001
EF Symptom Count—Short Form	2.0	3.2	6.6	5.0	23.37	< .001

Note. ODD, oppositional defiant disorder; F = results for the F-test; p, probability value for the F-test if ≤ .05; Self-Organization, Self-Organization/Problem Solving subscale; Self-Reg. of Emotion, Self-Regulation of Emotion subscale.

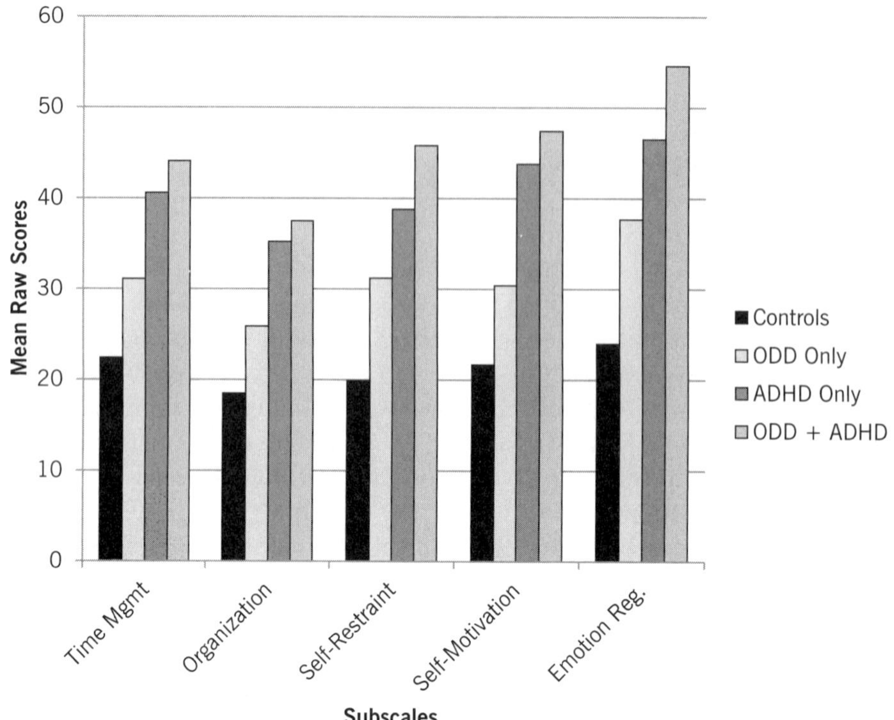

FIGURE 7.16. Raw scores for the BDEFS-CA subscales for children who had received a professional diagnosis of oppositional defiant disorder (ODD) alone, those with ADHD alone, having both disorders (ODD + ADHD), and the remainder of the sample (controls). Time Mgmt, Self-Management to Time subscale; Organization, Self-Organization/Problem Solving subscale; Emotion Reg., Self-Regulation of Emotion subscale.

than the control group as well, even if lower than those of the group with ADHD only. This suggests that some deficits in EF in daily life are associated with ODD, albeit far less severe than those seen in ADHD. However, on three of the scales, both of the ADHD groups had higher scores than either the ODD-only or control groups. On these three scales (Self-Management to Time, Self-Organization/Problem Solving, and Self-Motivation), the two ADHD groups did not differ from each other. On the two remaining scales (Self-Restraint and Self-Regulation of Emotion), there was evidence for complete separation among all four groups: ODD + ADHD > ADHD only > ODD only > controls. This suggests that the presence of comorbidity between these two disorders worsens these domains of EF in daily life beyond that seen in ADHD alone.

Given the small sample size, these findings can be tested again by a different approach to see whether these results still hold true, as was done earlier for BPD. When the entire ODD group is compared with the remainder of the sample using ANOVA but removing ADHD symptom severity as a covariate, the results show that there are no group differences on the same three subscales that also seemed to be unaffected by ODD, thus corroborating that result. The two subscales on which ODD seemed to have some effect remained significantly different in these reanalyses, thereby corroborating the original findings. This pattern is similar to the finding by Qian and colleagues (2010) for Chinese children in which the comorbid group scored worse on the BRIEF ratings than the ADHD-only group. It is also consistent with the view that ODD is most closely associated with and may arise in part from the impulsive emotion and poor emotional self-regulation features of ADHD (Barkley, 2010). As before, these findings also speak to the validity of the BDEFS-CA, just as was found for all other disorders discussed herein.

Patterns of EF Deficits within and across Disorders

It is possible to take the results from the tables in this chapter for each disorder and compute effect sizes (Cohen's *d*; Cohen, 1992) to create a common metric on which to compare them. It also permits us to obtain some idea of which disorders are most likely to disrupt which domains of EF in daily life and to what degree relative to the other disorders. This gives a picture of the pattern of EF deficits across disorders and within each disorder, allowing scores on all scales to be compared directly with each other by this standard metric (effect size). An effect size here is the difference in the mean raw scores between each disorder and the control group divided by the pooled standard deviation (for both the disordered and control groups). It is therefore the number of standard deviations that separate the mean scores for the disorder from the general population sample not having that disorder. Because ADHD has such a pervasive and substantial impact on EF in daily life activities in all domains, and because it can be comorbid with each of these disorders in a significant proportion of cases, those comorbid cases involving ADHD are removed from these analyses—except, of course, for the findings for ADHD itself.

In Table 7.19 one can see the effect size differences for each disorder on each of the five subscales of the BDEFS-CA. The effect sizes reflect just what would likely be associated with each disorder in the absence of empirically diagnosed cases of ADHD. Typically, an effect size of 0.20 is considered small, one of 0.50 is medium, and one of 0.80 is large (Cohen, 1992). The table also shows whether or not the disorder cases were significantly different from the control group when the pairwise comparisons were conducted ($p \leq .05$) between the disorder-only groups and the control groups. Again, all cases of ADHD were removed from these comparisons. Finally, and perhaps most clinically informative, this table also shows the percentage of cases of each disorder that placed in the clinically deficient range on each of the subscales (the rows are highlighted in bold in the table). The clinically deficient range is defined here (and traditionally) as having a score at or above the 93rd percentile for the individual's age group (6–11 or 12–17 years) and sex. Just 7% (approximately) of the population would expect to be in this range, which essentially places the participant 1.5 *SD* above the mean for the general population. Therefore, percentages for each disorder that are higher than 7% indicate that the disorder is associated with an elevation in risk of clinical deficiency on that subscale.

(text resumes on page 114)

TABLE 7.19. Comparison of BDEFS-CA Long Form Scores for Children with Various Developmental, Learning, and Psychiatric Disorders

Disorder[a]	Time Mgmt.	Self-Organize	Self-Restraint	Self-Motivate	Emotion Regulation
Attention-deficit/hyperactivity disorder (parent rated)					
ES	1.32	0.99	1.26	1.35	1.04
Magnitude[b]	Large	Large	Large	Large	Large
Significant[c]	Yes	Yes	Yes	Yes	Yes
% Deficient[d]	**43.4%**	**32.9%**	**43.9%**	**42.2%**	**34.1%**
Attention-deficit/hyperactivity disorder (research diagnosis)					
ES	2.48	1.93	2.48	2.86	2.16
Magnitude	X-large	X-large	X-large	X-large	X-large
Significant	Yes	Yes	Yes	Yes	Yes
% Deficient	**72.8%**	**68.0%**	**73.6%**	**77.6%**	**67.2%**
Speech and language disorders					
ES	0.26	0.63	0.21	0.40	0.27
Magnitude	Small	Medium	Small	Small	Small
Significant	No	Yes	No	Yes	No
% Deficient	**2.8%**	**19.4%**	**6.9%**	**9.7%**	**9.7%**
Developmental coordination disorder					
ES	0.43	0.87	0.45	0.66	0.46
Magnitude	Small	Large	Small	Medium	Small
Significant	Yes	Yes	Yes	Yes	Yes
% Deficient	**10.0%**	**27.5%**	**10.0%**	**7.5%**	**7.5%**
Developmental disability/mental retardation					
ES	0.77	1.46	0.71	1.16	0.91
Magnitude	Medium	Large	Medium	Large	Large
Significant	Yes	Yes	Yes	Yes	Yes
% Deficient	**22.2%**	**55.6%**	**11.1%**	**11.1%**	**11.1%**
Seizures/epilepsy					
ES	0.59	1.02	0.41	0.54	0.34
Magnitude	Medium	Large	Small	Medium	Small
Significant	No	Yes	No	Yes	No
% Deficient	**16.7%**	**41.7%**	**25.0%**	**25.0%**	**16.7%**
Tic disorder/Tourette syndrome					
ES	0.73	0.93	0.98	0.86	1.40
Magnitude	Medium	Large	Large	Large	Large
Significant	Yes	Yes	Yes	Yes	Yes
% Deficient	**12.5%**	**12.5%**	**25.0%**	**0.0%**	**37.5%**
Autism spectrum disorders					
ES	0.36	1.14	0.87	0.51	1.05
Magnitude	Small	Large	Large	Medium	Large
Significant	No	Yes	Yes	Yes	Yes
% Deficient	**0.0%**	**31.6%**	**36.8%**	**15.8%**	**21.1%**
Reading disorders					
ES	0.55	0.80	0.33	0.72	0.37
Magnitude	Medium	Large	Small	Medium	Small
Significant	Yes	Yes	No	Yes	No
% Deficient	**11.1%**	**16.7%**	**13.0%**	**13.0%**	**5.6%**

(cont.)

TABLE 7.19. *(cont.)*

Disorder[a]	Time Mgmt.	Self-Organize	Self-Restraint	Self-Motivate	Emotion Regulation
Spelling disorders					
ES	0.69	0.75	0.44	0.83	0.54
Magnitude	Medium	Medium	Small	Large	Medium
Significant	Yes	Yes	No	Yes	Yes
% Deficient	**9.1%**	**15.2%**	**6.1%**	**18.2%**	**3.0%**
Math disorders					
ES	0.87	1.16	0.38	1.07	0.55
Magnitude	Large	Large	Small	Large	Medium
Significant	Yes	Yes	No	Yes	Yes
% Deficient	**20.7%**	**27.6%**	**13.8%**	**20.7%**	**6.9%**
Writing disorders					
ES	0.80	1.11	0.65	1.05	0.68
Magnitude	Large	Large	Medium	Large	Medium
Significant	Yes	Yes	Yes	Yes	Yes
% Deficient	**14.3%**	**32.1%**	**14.3%**	**25.0%**	**7.1%**
Anxiety disorders					
ES	0.50	0.45	0.37	0.52	0.81
Magnitude	Medium	Small	Small	Medium	Large
Significant	Yes	Yes	No	Yes	Yes
% Deficient	**8.8%**	**8.8%**	**8.8%**	**11.8%**	**17.6%**
Depression					
ES	1.01	0.64	0.74	0.92	1.14
Magnitude	Large	Medium	Medium	Large	Large
Significant	Yes	Yes	Yes	Yes	Yes
% Deficient	**17.4%**	**21.7%**	**13.0%**	**21.7%**	**26.1%**
Oppositional defiant disorder					
ES	1.34	1.25	1.80	1.10	1.49
Magnitude	Large	Large	X-large	Large	Large
Significant	Yes	Yes	Yes	Yes	Yes
% Deficient	**18.2%**	**27.3%**	**36.4%**	**9.1%**	**36.4%**
Bipolar disorder					
ES	1.38	1.10	1.63	1.21	1.92
Magnitude	Large	Large	X-large	Large	X-large
Significant	Yes	Yes	Yes	Yes	Yes
% Deficient	**14.3%**	**14.3%**	**28.6%**	**28.6%**	**57.1%**

Note. ES = effect size (Cohen's *d*); research diagnosis, ADHD diagnosed by the research criteria reported in this manual (93rd percentile on ADHD symptom ratings and impairment in at least one domain); Time Mgmt, Self-Management to Time subscale; Self-Organize = Self-Organization/Problem Solving subscale; Self-Motivate, Self-Motivation subscale; Emotion Regulation, Self-Regulation of Emotion subscale.

[a]Except for ADHD, all disorders are based on parent-report of the child having received a professional diagnosis of that disorder. ADHD was also diagnosed by the research criteria presented in this manual (see above). All disorders except ADHD also have cases with comorbid ADHD (research diagnosis) removed from these analyses.

[b]Magnitude is graded as .20+ = small, .50+ = medium, .80+ = large (see Cohen, 1992), and 1.5+ = extra large (X-large).

[c]"Significant" means that the comparison between this disorder and the control group (both without ADHD cases) was significantly different from the remainder of the sample at $p < .05$.

[d]"% Deficient" means the percentage of children with this disorder who placed at or above the 93rd percentile for the normative sample ($N = 1,800$) for their age group (6–11 years, 12–17 years) and sex.

One can see very quickly from these three indicators (effect size, significance, and percentage deficient) what the impact is of each disorder on each domain of EF in daily life, controlling for cases of comorbidity with ADHD. The results are quite informative and, to my knowledge, exist nowhere else in the scientific literature on these disorders or on any parent rating scale of EF deficits. Bear in mind that the absolute number for the effect size here is not so important. It might well be different had a more rigorous approach to diagnosing these childhood disorders been used instead of parent reports of a professional diagnosis of their child. It is the *relative* pattern of effect sizes or deficits that is most informative here when comparing disorders with each other, as well as among the EF domains for any specific disorder.

The results show that ADHD has, by far, the most adverse effect on all domains of EF in daily life activities, regardless of which indicator is used. Whether it is based on parent-reported diagnosis by a professional or on the more rigorous research criteria used in this manual, ADHD results in far more severe effects on EF domains and in the inclusion of far more cases in the clinically deficient range than any other disorder. Indeed, using more rigorous criteria results in effect sizes about twice as large as those associated with parent-reported diagnoses, which placed well above the "large" designation of an EF. Using research criteria to define ADHD almost doubles the percentage of cases considered clinically deficient. This is most likely the result of the fact that professional diagnoses included cases of ADD, or the inattentive type of ADHD and perhaps even those of sluggish cognitive tempo (SCT), which may be a different disorder of attention, as noted in Chapter 4. In virtually every EF domain, the adverse effect of ADHD (research diagnosis) is 2–3 *SD* above the control mean; this effect size is not just large by traditional definition (Cohen, 1992) but huge. The findings essentially mean that the distributions of these scores for the ADHD group overlap minimally, if at all, with the remaining population of children. Indeed, as measured by effect sizes, the impact of ADHD is 2–11 times greater in each domain than is the case for any other disorder. This cannot be attributed to the possibility that the BDEFS-CA contains as many symptoms of ADHD as described in DSM-IV. Those symptoms were intentionally not included in the BDEFS or BDEFS-CA to permit the study of EF deficits in ADHD without such contamination of the dependent measure (EF) with the independent variable of interest (ADHD). Notice that the use of research diagnostic criteria also results in far more cases of ADHD placing in the clinically deficient range—the vast majority of ADHD cases are deficient in one or more of the BDEFS-CA subscales by that approach to diagnosis.

Not surprisingly, both ODD and BPD are the next most adverse disorders in their effects on EF in daily life across all domains on the BDEFS-CA as measured by effect sizes, but especially on Self-Regulation of Emotion. To understand why, consider that even after removing cases of ADHD diagnosed by research criteria, some variation in ADHD symptoms is still present within the remaining sample for that other disorder. Given the strong correlation of ADHD symptom severity with those of ODD and BDP (indeed, some symptoms of ADHD occur on the BPD symptom list), it is likely that the remaining variation in ADHD symptoms may be driving even these differences between ODD or BPD and the control group, or at least a portion of them. Recall from the previous discussion that when ADHD severity was covaried out of the group comparisons of the entire ODD group and the remainder of the sample, significant effects were evident only for the Self-Restraint and the Self-Regulation of Emotion subscales. This demonstrates that the large effect sizes seen in Table 7.19 for ODD for the remaining scales are likely due to its close association with severity of ADHD. These differences become nonsignificant when ADHD is entirely statistically removed from those comparisons. The same occurred for BPD when ADHD was covaried. Results for the Self-Management to Time and Self-Motivation domains became nonsignificant, whereas those effects for Self-Organization/Problem Solving, Self-Restraint, and Self-Regulation of Emotion remained significant. Looking at the percentage of cases in the clinically deficient range also tells us that although ODD and BPD are associated with some elevations on each subscale, the vast majority of children with ODD or BPD are not so deficient. The subscale with the greatest such deficient cases is Self-Regulation of Emotion, which makes perfect sense when one understands that ODD and BPD involve mood dysregulation, particularly for anger, hostility, and even aggression in the case of ODD (Barkley, 2010; Pliszka, 2009).

The problem of contamination of each disorder by subclinical levels of ADHD symptoms may even exist for some other disorders with which ADHD has a strong relationship. For instance, as noted, recent research suggests a shared genetic liability for ADHD, ASD, and DCD (not to mention ODD). It is therefore possible that some of the impact of these disorders on EF, as seen in Table 7.19, apart from ADHD, is still a reflection of variation of ADHD symptoms within these groups, albeit at less clinically significant levels. One should therefore consider even these effect sizes for the various non-ADHD disorders to be at a maximum, as they can still have some contamination with ADHD severity. That is the reason for the previous cautionary statement that it is the *relative* patterns of deficits here and not their absolute degree that is informative. It is also the reason that it is more helpful clinically to study the percentage of cases of each disorder that placed in the clinically deficient range.

But there is also some good reason to expect that each of these disorders may have a negative impact on certain cognitive components of EF, as discussed. Those would translate into some degree of adverse effect on the parent-rated EF domain in daily life most related to it and when independent of ADHD, such as between language and self-organization and problem solving. That is the reason that the pairwise comparisons reported for each disorder alone as against those involving comorbidity with ADHD may be as or more revealing of the impact of that disorder on EF than are the results for the effect sizes shown in Table 7.19. Even more clinically informative, again, is that percentage of cases placing in the clinically deficient range on each subscale.

Some patterns here are quite surprising. Consider the case of TD/TS, for which, as noted, research had suggested that EF deficits as assessed by psychometric tests were largely if not entirely related to the comorbidity of ADHD with these movement disorders. The present results indicate that this is not the case, as those disorders were associated with large effect size differences across all five domains of the BDEFS-CA. Such results are in agreement with at least one study (see earlier discussion) that also used a rating scale of EF deficits and found significantly elevated scores for cases of this disorder. These and other results suggest the possibility that EF ratings may be more sensitive to the EF deficits related to various disorders than are EF tests. Given the low and often nonsignificant relationship of EF tests to EF ratings discussed here and in Chapter 1, it is clear that these two different approaches to measurement are not assessing the same construct. It is also becoming increasingly obvious that EF ratings are far more predictive of impairment in major life activities and adaptive functioning than are EF tests. By these criteria, EF ratings may therefore be a more valid index of EF deficits than are the more frequently used and much venerated EF tests. Returning to TD/TS, it is noteworthy that despite large effect size differences from the control group across the EF subscales, the vast majority of children with these disorders did not place in the clinically deficient range on the EF subscales. The greatest percentage of cases fell on the scales on which one would expect for such disorders of inhibition—the Self-Restraint and Self-Regulation of Emotion subscales.

Now look at the various learning disabilities, whether reading, spelling, math, language, or writing disorders. The evidence from effect sizes tells us that these disorders are associated with a small impact on EF in daily life across these domains, and particularly so for Self-Organization/Problem Solving. Yet when one examines the proportion of cases that would likely fall in the clinically deficient range on any BDEFS-CA subscales, it is clear that the vast majority of cases are unlikely to do so. It is of interest that math and writing disorders seem to have a greater adverse association with EF domains than do reading, spelling, and speech/language disorders. The reason for this is unclear.

Another interesting finding has to do with anxiety disorders. Notice that once ADHD cases have been removed, anxiety disorders have only a modest adverse effect on the EF subscales as indexed by effect sizes. Yet even this is not especially impressive when translated into the percentage of cases that are likely to be clinically deficient on any subscales, as the proportion is barely above that expected from the population average of 7% for most scales (8–11%). The only elevation in risk from anxiety disorders seems to be on the Self-Regulation of Emotion scale, as one might expect from the very nature of this class of child psychiatric disorders. In contrast, the adverse impact of depression on EF in daily life is significantly greater, resulting in an approximately twofold increase in risk of being clinically deficient in each of the EF subscale domains. Once again, as would be expected from the nature of this mood disorder, the greatest impact of depression is in the domain of Self-Regulation of Emotion.

Looking down each column in Table 7.19 shows that different disorders have a clearly different degree of adverse relationship with deficits in that EF domain. For example, under the "Time Mgmt" domain (Self-Regulation to Time), it is ADHD, followed by ODD and then depression, that has the most adverse impact on this domain. ASD and BPD, on the other hand, seem to have little or no relationship to this domain once ADHD cases have been removed. In contrast, under the Self-Restraint domain, one finds again that ADHD is linked to the greatest level of deficits. This is hardly surprising considering that poor inhibition is a central feature of this disorder (Barkley, 1997a). The disorder with the next greatest impact on that EF domain is again ODD, followed by BPD and then TD/TS. Most of these disorders are thought to involve difficulties with impulse control or self-restraint, and that is reflected in these findings. The pattern of effect sizes for Self-Organization/Problem Solving shows the following order for the disorders ranked highest in adverse effects on this domain: ADHD > DD/MR > ODD > BPD. Using the metric of the percentage of cases that are clinically deficient, the pattern now includes ADHD > DD/MR > seizure disorders > ASD. The small number of cases of seizure disorders may have contributed to this change in patterns simply because each case carries a greater weight in computing the percentages.

Inspecting the column for Self-Motivation, and especially using the metric of percentage clinically deficient, shows just as curious and interesting a pattern as with Self-Management to Time. ADHD, again, is associated with the greatest risk, whereas speech/language, motor, DD/MR, TD/TS, anxiety, and ODD have almost no elevation of risk in this EF domain. And the risk associated with the other disorders, such as those of reading, spelling, and math, is not that much higher than the base rate of the population. Next to ADHD, most other disorders pale in their clinical impact on this domain. This is understandable given that theories of ADHD have often stressed that it involves an inherent problem with self-motivation (Barkley, 1997a, 1997c) or sensitivity to reinforcement, particularly under schedules of delayed consequences (Haenlein & Caul, 1987; Luman, Oosterlaan, & Sergeant, 2005). A similar conclusion can be reached about the results for the next domain of EF, the Self-Regulation of Emotion. Here one finds that disorders that ought to have the greatest adverse association with this domain of EF in fact do so. These are ADHD, ODD, depression, and BPD.

These findings are not just incredibly informative concerning the specific disorders and their differential effects on the specific domains of EF in daily life; they are a clear testament to the criterion validity of the BDEFS-CA and its ability to discern different patterns of adverse effects across different disorders, as one might expect given what is known about the nature of these various disorders. Certainly these results are not definitive given the limitations of this study: (1) reliance on parental report of diagnoses, except in ADHD; (2) small sample sizes in some cells of the analyses, especially after removing comorbid ADHD cases, thus limiting statistical power to detect less than large effect sizes as significant; and (3) the difficulties in exploring two- and three-way comorbidities for their impact on EF in daily life. These limitations provide ample justification, if more were needed, to further explore these issues with larger samples of better diagnosed cases than was possible here. Yet this is a reasonable initial step toward doing so. It also provided substantial evidence for the validity of the BDEFS-CA.

Conclusion

This chapter has provided a large body of evidence in support of the validity of the BDEFS-CA for evaluating EF in the daily life activities of children. Whether it is for construct, convergent, divergent, or criterion validity, the evidence is sufficient to validate this measure of EF in daily life. The most clinically and scientifically informative evidence for the utility of the BDEFS-CA comes from the abundant evidence herein that it can readily distinguish various patterns of EF deficits in daily life across various neurodevelopmental, learning, and psychiatric disorders of childhood. It does so beyond the far easier task of just differentiating between various disordered groups and a control group not having that disorder. Evidence here also makes it clear that ADHD has the most severe and pervasive impact on EF in daily life activities, adversely affecting all domains to a substantial degree. Therefore, it was important to remove such cases when comparing disorders with each other and with control groups given that ADHD is known to be a significant comorbid condition for the vast majority of the disorders discussed here. When that was done, interesting and distinct patterns of impairment in various domains of EF were evident across the disorders. Such evidence shows that the BDEFS-CA has considerable utility both in clinical practice, in which cases of such disorders must be evaluated, and also in research into the nature of EF deficits in these disorders. The results here lend confidence that more rigorous investigations into the nature of EF deficits in these disorders are likely to be revealing, rewarded, and worthwhile.

The next chapter reviews another line of evidence for the validity of the BDEFS-CA—its relationship to various measures of impairment in daily life collected on this large general population sample of children. This is yet more evidence for the criterion validity of the BDEFS-CA, and it is also evidence of its ecological validity in showing associations between the scale scores and various indicators of impaired functioning in major domains of life activities for children.

CHAPTER 8

Relationship of BDEFS-CA Scores to Impairment

This chapter provides further evidence for the criterion and ecological validity of the BDEFS-CA scores by examining their relationship to various measures of impairment collected on the entire original sample. As has been noted previously (Barkley, 2011b), symptoms and impairments are not identical and do not have a perfectly direct relationship to each other. Symptoms can be viewed as the cognitions and behaviors associated with and arising from a particular disorder. Impairments are the consequences those cognitions and behaviors have in the person's life. The items on the BDEFS-CA can be largely if not entirely conceptualized as symptoms of deficient EF. This chapter examines the relationship of such symptoms to the consequences that ensue as a result of variation in the severity of those EF symptoms. I begin with an obvious domain of consequences: the extent to which the children in the sample have been treated with psychiatric, educational, and psychological therapies. Is the extent of each of these treatments in any way related to the severity of EF symptoms as reflected across the BDEFS-CA subscales?

Relationship to Treatments

One obvious consequence or outcome that may be associated with having EF deficits is the extent to which the child has been given psychiatric medications. There is every reason to suspect just such a relationship given the findings in the previous chapter: EF deficits are found in conjunction with many psychiatric and developmental disorders, and psychiatric medications are often used to treat such disorders, especially ADHD. Parents in the sample were asked if their children had ever been treated with psychiatric medications for management of a psychiatric or psychological disorder. Children who had been treated were compared with those not treated on all 10 of the BDEFS-CA scores. The results are shown in Table 8.1, in which it is evident that all ANOVAs were significant at $p < .001$. A more informative means of conveying this relationship in seeking evidence for the validity of the BDEFS-CA subscale scores is to consider what percentage of children who had placed in the clinically deficient range on the BDEFS-CA subscales were treated with psychiatric medications compared to the remainder of the original sample. The results appear in Figure 8.1 where one can see that children falling in the clinically deficient range on any given subscale were six to seven times more likely to have been treated with a psychiatric medication than children not in the deficient range (all χ^2's had p's $< .001$). This finding is not so surprising when one considers that 41 percent of individuals who received a research diagnosis of ADHD (and 65% of those with parent-reported professional diagnoses of ADHD or ADD) were being treated with medication and that ADHD has the greatest adverse relationship with EF deficits in daily life activities. The next most likely disorders among those receiving medication were anxiety disorders (23.1%) and depression (10.2%).

Parents also reported on the educational treatments their children had received. The results for those reporting that their children had received some type of formal academic tutoring are shown in Table 8.2. All of the comparisons were statistically significant at $p < .001$. Children who had received tutoring had significantly higher scores on all of the BDEFS-CA scores. Again, examining the reverse relationship, one can ask whether those who had received clinically elevated (deficient) ratings on the BDEFS-CA subscales were more likely to be receiving such tutoring. The answer is clearly affirmative, as shown in Figure 8.2, which shows that children who

TABLE 8.1 BDEFS-CA Long and Short Form scores for Children Who Had and Had Not Received Psychiatric Medication

	No medication (N= 1,766)		Medication (N= 156)			
Subscale	Mean	*SD*	Mean	*SD*	*F*	*p*
Self-Management to Time	22.7	8.1	34.0	10.1	266.80	< .001
Self-Organization	18.8	6.5	28.3	11.7	257.68	< .001
Self-Restraint	20.3	7.5	31.8	10.9	306.49	< .001
Self-Motivation	22.2	8.7	34.7	11.7	279.59	< .001
Self-Reg. of Emotion	24.4	9.6	39.1	14.2	305.88	< .001
Total EF Summary Score	108.5	35.3	167.9	50.4	374.64	< .001
ADHD-EF Index	14.8	4.8	22.7	7.2	349.10	< .001
EF Symptom Count	7.1	12.6	29.9	21.5	403.80	< .001
EF Summary Score—Short Form	31.8	10.3	49.1	14.4	374.78	< .001
EF Symptom Count—Short Form	2.3	3.8	9.0	6.3	395.37	< .001

Note. *F*, results for the *F*-test; *p*, probability value for the *F*-test if ≤ .05; Self-Organization, Self-Organization/Problem Solving subscale; Self-Reg. of Emotion, Self-Regulation of Emotion subscale.

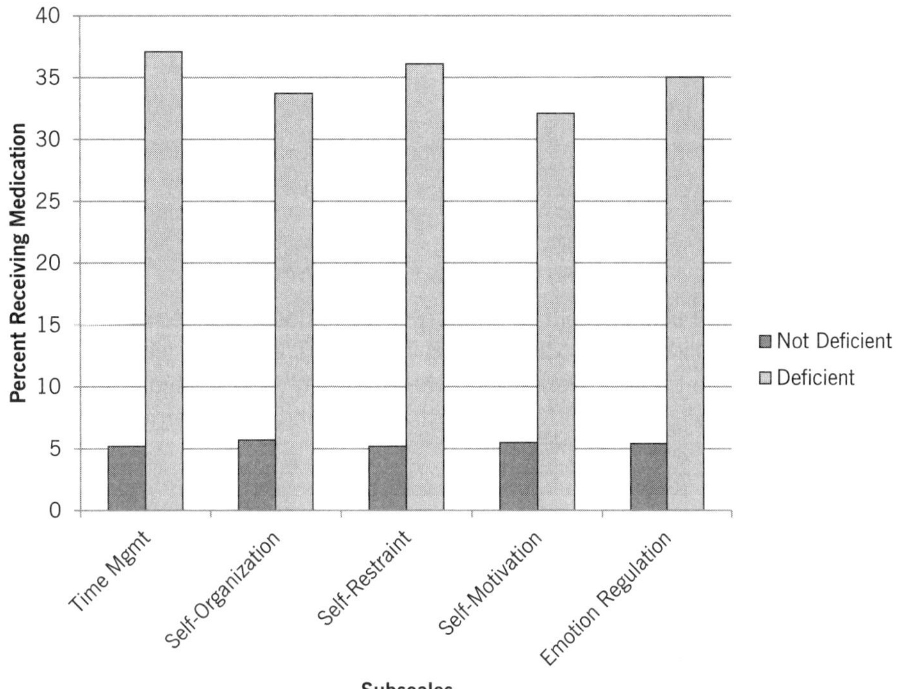

FIGURE 8.1. Percentage of children placing in the clinically deficient range (≥ 93rd percentile) or not deficient on each BDEFS-CA subscale who had received a psychiatric medication. All comparisons are significant at $p < .001$. Time Mgmt, Self-Management to Time subscale; Self-Organization, Self-Organization/Problem Solving subscale; Emotion Regulation, Self-Regulation of Emotion subscale.

TABLE 8.2. BDEFS-CA Long and Short Form Scores for Children Who Had and Had Not Received Formal Academic Tutoring

	No tutoring (N = 1,842)		Tutoring (N = 80)			
Subscale	Mean	*SD*	Mean	*SD*	*F*	*p*
Self-Management to Time	23.3	8.6	30.1	10.8	45.61	< .001
Self-Organization	19.3	7.2	26.4	11.3	71.21	< .001
Self-Restraint	21.0	8.2	26.8	11.2	35.91	< .001
Self-Motivation	22.8	9.3	31.2	12.4	59.19	< .001
Self-Reg. of Emotion	25.2	10.5	33.4	14.3	44.52	< .001
Total EF Summary Score	111.8	38.8	147.9	53.6	63.70	< .001
ADHD-EF Index	15.2	5.3	20.4	7.5	68.75	< .001
EF Symptom Count	8.4	14.3	21.4	21.5	56.51	< .001
EF Summary Score—Short Form	32.8	11.2	43.5	15.5	66.46	< .001
EF Symptom Count—Short Form	2.6	6.6	4.3	6.3	61.82	< .001

Note. F, results for the F-test; p, probability value for the F-test if ≤ .05; Self-Organization, Self-Organization/Problem Solving subscale; Self-Reg. of Emotion, Self-Regulation of Emotion subscale.

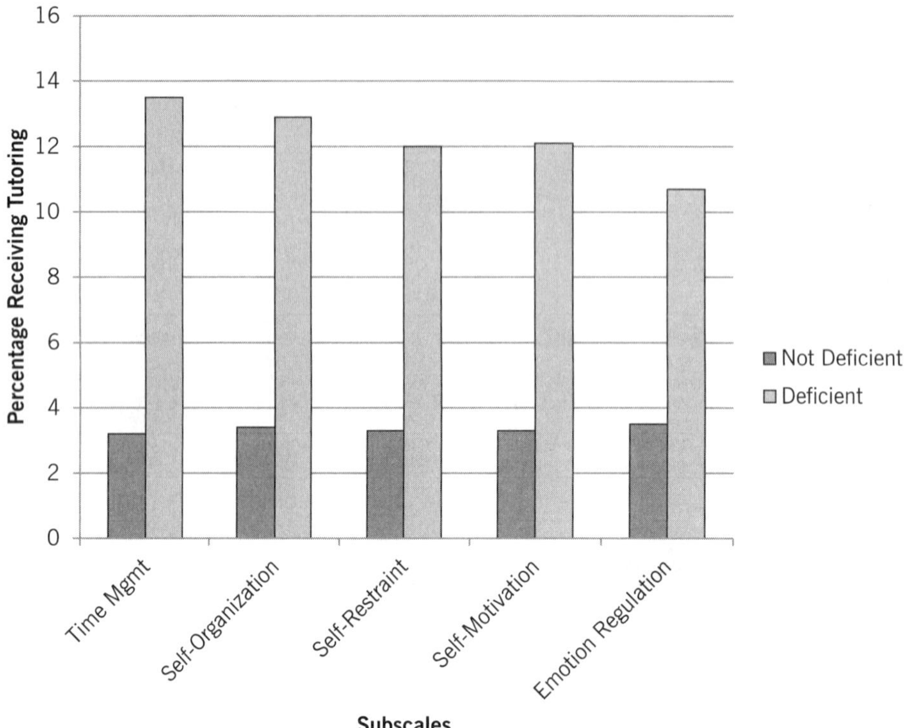

FIGURE 8.2. Percentage of children placing in the clinically deficient range (≥ 93rd percentile) or not deficient on each BDEFS-CA subscale who had received formal academic tutoring. All comparisons are significant at $p < .001$. Time Mgmt, Self-Management to Time subscale; Self-Organization, Self-Organization/Problem Solving subscale; Emotion Regulation, Self-Regulation of Emotion subscale.

placed in that clinical range on the BDEFS-CA subscales were four to six times more likely to have received such services (all χ^2's had p's < .001).

Academic assistance may also be given in the form of special education services at school. Children who were reported by parents to have received special education were compared with those who had not on all 10 BDEFS-CA scores. Those results appear in Table 8.3. All comparisons were again significant at $p < .001$. As above, the children who had received formal special education had higher scores on all scores of the scale compared with those who did not receive such services. Again taking the alternative view, one can examine the percentage of children receiving high scores on the subscales that placed them in the clinically deficient range compared with those who did not place in that range and who received such educational services. These results are shown graphically in Figure 8.3. They make it clear that children in the clinically deficient range on the BDEFS-CA subscales were five to six times more likely to have received special education services at school (all χ^2's had p's < .001).

Precisely the same pattern of findings was evident for children who had received speech and language therapy at school ($N = 219$). Those who had received such therapy had significantly higher scores on the BDEFS-CA scores than did those

TABLE 8.3. BDEFS-CA Long and Short Form Scores for Children Who Had and Had Not Received Special Education Services at School

	No special education (N= 1,746)		Special education (N= 176)			
Subscale	Mean	*SD*	Mean	*SD*	*F*	*p*
Self-Management to Time	22.7	8.2	32.3	9.9	207.26	< .001
Self-Organization	18.7	6.6	28.1	10.2	283.92	< .001
Self-Restraint	20.5	7.7	29.3	10.7	194.54	< .001
Self-Motivation	22.1	8.8	33.6	11.2	258.05	< .001
Self-Reg. of Emotion	24.6	9.9	35.1	13.8	164.22	< .001
Total EF Summary Score	108.7	36.4	158.5	47.4	281.05	< .001
ADHD-EF Index	14.8	4.9	21.8	6.7	301.61	< .001
EF Symptom Count	7.2	13.1	25.7	20.7	280.13	< .001
EF Summary Score—Short Form	31.9	10.6	46.2	13.7	274.92	< .001
EF Symptom Count—Short Form	2.3	3.9	7.6	6.1	259.93	< .001

Note. F, results for the *F*-test; *p*, probability value for the *F*-test if ≤ .05; Self-Organization, Self-Organization/Problem Solving subscale; Self-Reg. of Emotion, Self-Regulation of Emotion subscale.

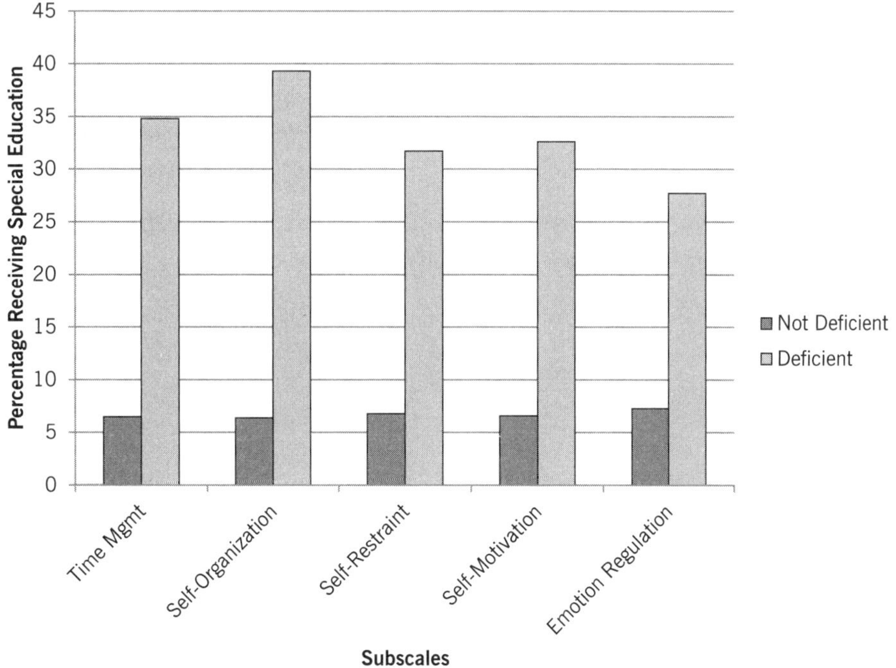

FIGURE 8.3. Percentage of children placing in the clinically deficient range (≥ 93rd percentile) or not deficient on each BDEFS-CA subscale who had received formal special education services at school. All comparisons are significant at $p < .001$. Time Mgmt, Self-Management to Time subscale; Self-Organization, Self-Organization/Problem Solving subscale; Emotion Regulation, Self-Regulation of Emotion subscale.

who had not (N = 1,703; all p's < .001). And again, the reverse relationship was also significant—those who placed in the clinically elevated range on the BDEFS-CA subscales were two to four times more likely to have received such services: Self-Management to Time (25.3 vs. 10%, respectively); Self-Organization/Problem Solving (33.1 vs. 9.4%), Self-Restraint (24 vs. 10.1%), Self-Motivation (22.6 vs. 10.2%), and Self-Regulation of Emotion (22.6 vs. 10.3%; all χ^2's had p's < .001). Similar results were evident for those who had received occupational therapy services (N = 85) compared with those who had not (N = 1,837) in that the former had significantly higher scores on all BDEFS-CA scores than those who did not. Also, those in the clinically deficient range on the BDEFS-CA subscales were four to seven times more likely to have had such services: Self-Management to Time (15.7 vs. 3.3%, respectively); Self-Organization/Problem Solving (21.5 vs. 2.8%), Self-Restraint (16.9 vs. 3.1%), Self-Motivation (12.6 vs. 3.5%), and Self-Regulation of Emotion (17.5 vs. 3.1%; all χ^2's had p's < .001). The situation was much the same for children who had received physical therapy services (N = 58) compared with those who had not (N = 1,864; all p's < .001). Yet again children in the clinically deficient range were two to three times more likely to have received such services (all χ^2's had p's < .005).

Parents reported that 187 children had received some type of individual psychological counseling or therapy. Compared with the scores of children who had not received such services, all 10 scores on the BDEFS-CA were significant at the p < .001 level. Those findings are shown in Table 8.4. As with all of the previous comparisons, it was also clear that children who placed in the clinically deficient range on the five subscales were five to ten times more likely to have received such counseling or therapy, as is evident in Figure 8.4. Results were essentially the same for those children who had and had not received family, group, or inpatient psychological

TABLE 8.4. BDEFS-CA Long and Short Form Scores for Children Who Had and Had Not Received Individual Psychological Counseling or Therapy

	No individual therapy (N = 1,735)		Individual therapy (N = 187)			
Subscale	Mean	*SD*	Mean	*SD*	*F*	*p*
Self-Management to Time	22.8	8.3	30.9	10.3	151.79	< .001
Self-Organization	19.1	7.0	24.4	10.0	86.54	< .001
Self-Restraint	20.4	7.7	29.4	10.7	210.75	< .001
Self-Motivation	22.3	8.9	31.6	12.0	172.29	< .001
Self-Reg. of Emotion	24.4	9.7	36.8	13.9	252.13	< .001
Total EF Summary Score	109.0	36.6	153.0	49.5	226.24	< .001
ADHD-EF Index	14.9	5.1	20.5	6.8	193.43	< .001
EF Symptom Count	7.3	13.1	24.2	20.9	245.36	< .001
EF Summary Score—Short Form	32.0	10.6	44.6	14.4	221.94	< .001
EF Symptom Count—Short Form	2.3	3.9	7.3	6.2	234.91	< .001

Note. F, results for the F-test; p, probability value for the F-test if ≤ .05; Self-Organization, Self-Organization/Problem Solving subscale; Self-Reg. of Emotion, Self-Regulation of Emotion subscale.

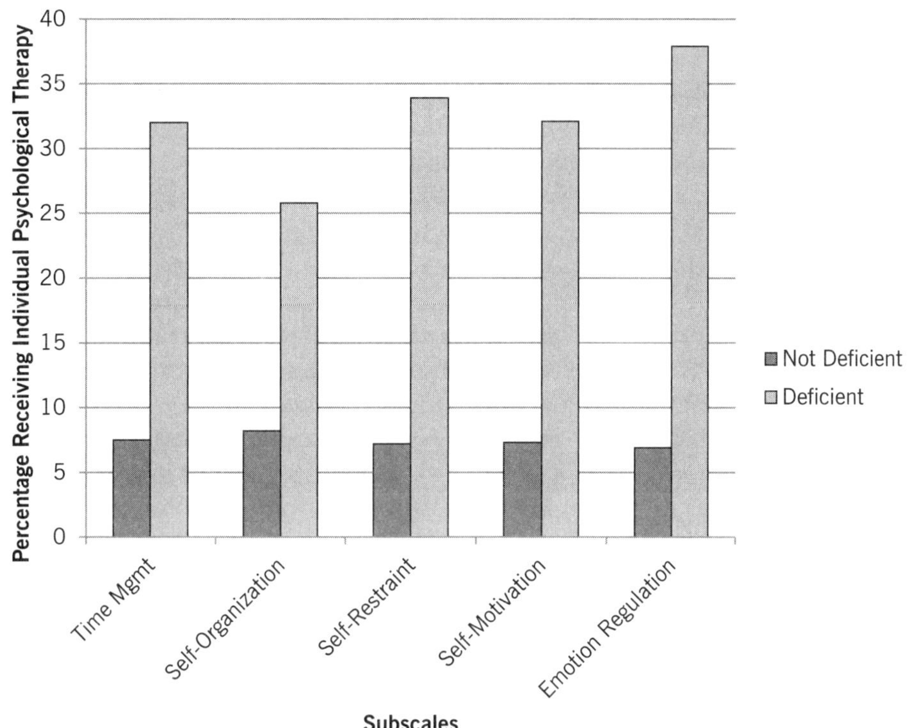

FIGURE 8.4. Percentage of children placing in the clinically deficient range (≥ 93rd percentile) or not deficient on each BDEFS-CA subscale who had received individual psychological therapy. All comparisons are significant at $p < .001$. Time Mgmt, Self-Management to Time subscale; Self-Organization, Self-Organization/Problem Solving subscale; Emotion Regulation, Self-Regulation of Emotion subscale.

treatment. And when comparing children in the clinically deficient range on the BDEFS-CA subscales, those in that range were 5 to 10 times more likely to have received each of these various services. Thus, to the extent that the receipt of treatment can be taken as a marker for impairment in major domains of life activities, numerous lines of evidence here indicate that children receiving such treatments have significantly higher scores on the BDEFS-CA and that those having clinically elevated BDEFS-CA subscale scores are far more likely to have received such treatments. No comparable evidence could be located about other EF rating scales for parents, such as the BRIEF, for comparison with these results (Gioia et al., 2000).

Ratings of Impairment

Impairment was assessed more directly in the original sample by having parents complete a rating scale assessing degree of psychosocial impairment in 15 domains of major life activities on the Barkley Functional Impairment Scale—Children and Adolescents (BFIS-CA; Barkley, 2012a). On this scale, each domain is rated on a 0 (*not at all*) to 9 (*severely impaired*) Likert scale. Parents also indicated whether any domain was not applicable to their child. Such responses were treated as missing data in the correlation analyses. These ratings of impairment were then correlated with the 10 BDEFS-CA scores as another indicator of criterion validity. The results for these Pearson product–moment correlations are shown in Table 8.5. All correlations were of a moderate magnitude and significant (all *p*'s < .001). The pattern of scores is informative and provides yet more evidence of validity of the BDEFS-CA. Notice that the highest correlations in the table are between the various BDEFS-CA scores and those domains of impairment that one would expect would place heavier demands on EF (or self-regulation), such as school performance, following rules, doing chores, and school homework, in comparison with domains expected to be less taxing of EF, such as playing with other children, playing sports, or visiting others. And as might be expected, the highest correlations are between the EF Summary Score representing the entire EF construct and the various BFIS domains of impairment. Also noteworthy is the fact that the short form scores (last two columns, EFSF and SCSF) are as highly related to each domain of impairment as are their long form equivalents (columns EF and SC). Examining the column showing the relations of the EF Summary Score to each domain, one can see that the total

TABLE 8.5. Correlations of BDEFS-CA Long and Short Form Scores with Ratings on 15 Domains of Impairment from the BFIS-CA

	BDEFS-CA scores									
BFIS-CA domains	TM	SO	SR	SM	SRE	EF	ADHD	SC	EFSF	SCSF
With mother	.47	.40	.54	.50	.53	.56	.52	.55	.56	.55
With father	.46	.41	.49	.48	.50	.53	.50	.52	.53	.52
School performance	.61	.58	.59	.67	.53	.67	.66	.67	.66	.65
With siblings	.49	.49	.59	.54	.60	.62	.59	.60	.61	.60
With other children	.42	.51	.53	.50	.55	.57	.57	.56	.56	.55
Community act.	.44	.51	.50	.49	.50	.55	.55	.54	.54	.53
Visiting others	.43	.51	.49	.47	.47	.53	.54	.52	.52	.51
Playing at school	.47	.54	.54	.52	.54	.59	.59	.58	.58	.56
Managing money	.50	.50	.56	.55	.49	.58	.59	.58	.58	.56
Self-care	.46	.48	.46	.51	.42	.53	.53	.52	.52	.51
Doing chores	.67	.53	.61	.71	.55	.69	.66	.68	.68	.67
School homework	.67	.56	.60	.72	.52	.69	.67	.69	.68	.68
Following rules	.61	.55	.67	.68	.61	.70	.68	.70	.69	.69
With other adults	.44	.52	.51	.50	.51	.56	.57	.56	.55	.55
Playing sports	.41	.49	.47	.49	.49	.53	.53	.53	.51	.51

Note. Analyses: Pearson product–moment correlations. All correlations are significant at *p* < .001. Sample sizes for correlations range from 1,607 to 1,824. TM, Self-Management to Time subscale; SO, Self-Organization/Problem Solving; SR, Self-Restraint subscale; SM, Self-Motivation subscale; SRE, Self-Regulation of Emotion subscale; ADHD, ADHD-EF Index; SC, EF symptom count; EF, EF Summary Score; SCSF, EF symptom count from Short Form; EFSF, EF Summary Score from Short Form.

BDEFS-CA score from the long form shares from 28 to 49% of the variance with the impairment ratings. The results are similar to those found for the adult version of the BDEFS in its relationship to ratings of adult major life activities (Barkley, 2011a). Such findings provide even more evidence for the criterion validity of the BDEFS-CA.

Another approach to studying the relationship of the BDEFS-CA to impairment ratings is to compare those children who placed in the clinically deficient range (at or above the 93rd percentile for age group and sex) on the EF Summary Score from the long form with those children who were not so classified. These comparisons can be made on each of the 15 domain ratings from the BFIS-CA. Those comparisons appear in Table 8.6. All comparisons were significant ($p < .001$), and the results show that individuals placing in the clinically deficient range in overall EF deficits had impairment scores that averaged four to five times higher in each domain than did those not so categorized. Considering that most children had impairment ratings of just 0 or 1 in each domain, the mean impairment scores for the EF-deficient group are strikingly deviant.

Overall, these results provide important evidence for the criterion validity of the BDEFS-CA scores as being related to and predictive of degrees of impairment in psychosocial functioning in the most important domains of children's major life activities. The higher the BDEFS-CA scores are, the greater is the degree of impair-

TABLE 8.6. Total EF Summary Scores for Children Who Did or Did Not Place in the Clinically Deficient Range on the 15 Domains from the BFIS-CA

	Not EF deficient		EF deficient			
BFIS-CA domain	Mean	*SD*	Mean	*SD*	*F*	*p*
With mother	0.8	1.7	4.2	2.9	505.77	< .001
With father	0.9	1.8	4.2	2.9	409.92	< .001
School performance	1.0	1.9	5.6	2.6	774.69	< .001
With siblings	1.0	1.8	5.0	2.7	539.74	< .001
With other children	0.7	1.6	4.0	2.8	522.07	< .001
Community activities	0.6	1.4	3.6	2.9	441.75	< .001
Visiting others	0.6	1.4	3.3	2.8	426.95	< .001
Playing at school	0.7	1.5	4.0	2.9	571.12	< .001
Managing money	0.8	1.6	4.4	3.1	531.37	< .001
Self-care	0.6	1.4	3.5	3.1	432.78	< .001
Doing chores	1.3	1.8	5.8	2.7	832.43	< .001
School homework	1.2	1.9	5.8	2.7	783.40	< .001
Following rules	0.8	1.6	5.4	2.8	1082.64	< .001
With other adults	0.6	1.4	3.7	2.9	593.56	< .001
Playing sports	0.7	1.6	3.8	2.8	363.00	< .001

Note. F, results for the *F*-test; *p*, probability value for the *F*-test if ≤ .05.

ment a child will be likely to experience in these domains. These results cannot be directly compared with those from other EF rating scales, such as the BRIEF for parents, given that no results are provided for the relationship of the scale to measures of impairment (Gioia et al., 2000).

Specific Areas of Psychosocial Impairment

Parents in the original sample were asked questions about specific areas of important psychosocial adjustment as another indicator of potential impairment in their children. The relationship of these measures to BDEFS-CA scores is now examined for further evidence of validity.

Friendships

Parents were asked about the number of friends their children currently had. The range of friends was from 0 to 99, with a mean = 7.7 (*SD* = 8.4). The distribution was highly skewed, with most parents reporting that their children had from 3 to 10 friends, with the median and the mode both being 5. Correlations for the five BDEFS-CA subscale scores ranged from –.10 for Self-Organization/Problem Solving to –.13 for Self-Regulation of Emotion, with all correlations being significant at $p < .001$. The EF Summary Score correlated –.13 with this measure of friendships ($p < .001$). Similar results were obtained for the other scores from the long and short forms. Given the skew of this distribution, which can distort a correlation coefficient, a better way of portraying the relationship of the BDEFS-CA scores to this measure of impairment is to subdivide the sample into those having one or no friends and those with two or more. Having one or fewer friends represents the bottom 5.7% of the population sample. It could be taken as an index of impairment in friendships with other children and certainly as a marker for their being unpopular. This unpopular group comprised 108 children, and they were compared to the remainder of the sample on the 5 BDEFS-CA subscales. The results are shown graphically in Figure 8.5. All comparisons were significant ($p < .001$). Clearly, higher BDEFS-CA scores are associated with being in the unpopular group, especially on the Self-Regulation of Emotion scale. That makes sense given the importance of this EF domain for sustaining friendships with others. An alternative means of examining the relationship of BDEFS-CA scores to friendships is by evaluating the percentage of children placing in the clinically deficient range on the BDEFS-CA subscales who placed in the unpopular group. Results indicated that children in the deficient range on the subscales were three to four times more likely to place in the unpopular group than were children not in the deficient range: Self-Management to Time (16.9 vs. 4.5%, respectively); Self-Organization/Problem Solving (19.1 vs. 4.4%); Self-Restraint (19.2 vs. 4.2%); Self-Motivation (16.4 vs. 4.5%); and Self-Regulation of Emotion (15.9 vs. 4.6%; all χ^2's had *p*'s < .001). On average, children who placed in the clinically deficient range had two (Self-Organization/Problem Solving) to three (Self-Management to Time) fewer friends than those not falling in the deficient range (all comparisons significant at $p < .001$).

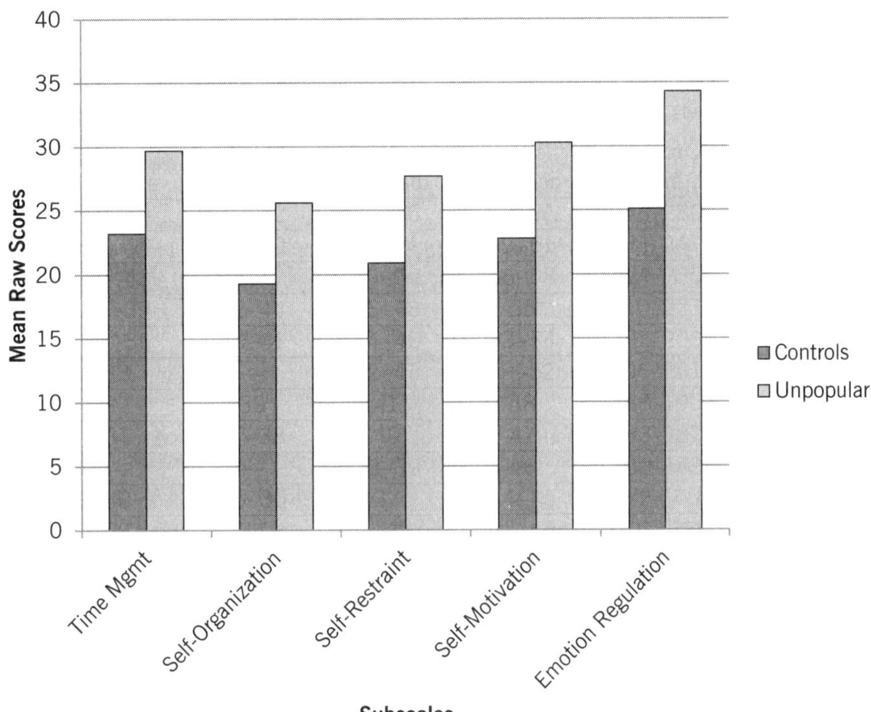

FIGURE 8.5. Mean raw scores for the five BDEFS-CA subscales for children who are unpopular (have one or no friends) and those in the control group (remainder of sample) who had at least two friends by parent report. All comparisons are significant at $p < .001$. Time Mgmt, Self-Management to Time subscale; Self-Organization, Self-Organization/Problem Solving subscale; Emotion Regulation, Self-Regulation of Emotion subscale.

Community Activities

Parents reported the number of clubs, sports, church groups, and organizations their children had belonged to in the previous year. The mean was 2.2 ($SD = 2.3$; median = 2; mode = 2). Eighty-nine percent of children belonged to 4 or fewer such community organizations. The correlations between the BDEFS-CA subscale scores ranged from –.11 (Self-Organization/Problem Solving) to –.17 (Self-Motivation), with all being significant at $p < .001$. The correlation for the EF Summary Score was –.15. There is a small but significant relationship between parent-reported EF deficits on the BDEFS-CA and the extent of involvement of children in various organized community activities. Parents were also asked about the number of formal organized sports in which their children participated in the past year apart from the physical education classes at school. The mean was 1.2 ($SD = 1.4$; median = 1; mode = 0). The correlations between the BDEFS-CA subscales and the sports participation ranged from –.10 (Self-Organization/Problem Solving) to –.15 (Self-Motivation), with the correlation of the EF Summary Score being –.14 (all p's < .001). As with clubs and other organized community activities, there is a small but significant negative relationship between EF deficits rated by parents and sports participation.

School Grades

Each parent in the original sample was asked to indicate his/her child's grade point average as reported on his/her previous report card using the following response categories: A (90–100%), B (80–89%), C (70–79%), D (60–69%), and E or F (50–59% or failing). 1,861 parents provided information to this question as follows: A, 54%, B, 32%, C, 11%, D, 2%, and F, 1%. The correlations between the BDEFS-CA subscale scores and this measure were: Self-Management to Time = –.44, Self-Organization/Problem Solving, –.38; Self-Restraint, –.35; Self-Motivation, –.47; Self-Regulation of Emotion, –.28; and EF Summary Score, –.43 (all p's < .001). The results were essentially of the same magnitude for the other BDEFS-CA scores from the long and short forms as for the EF Summary Score. Thus BDEFS-CA subscales share up to 22% of the variance with parental reports of their children's grade point averages. Another way of illustrating this relationship is to compare children who placed in the C or lower range of grades (14% of sample) with those who had A or B averages. This comparison is shown in Figure 8.6. All comparisons were significant at the $p < .001$ level. Obviously, children with higher grades have significantly lower BDEFS-CA subscale scores. This was also true for the Total EF Summary Score: A–B

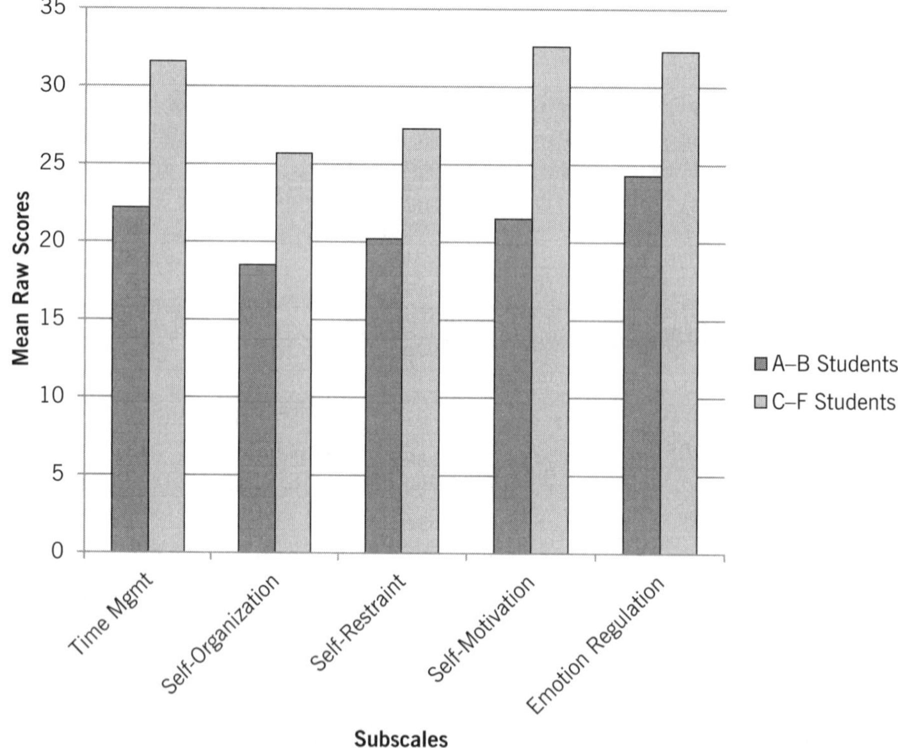

FIGURE 8.6. Mean raw scores for the five BDEFS-CA subscales for children who were reported by parents to be A or B students compared with those for children reported to be C, D, or F students on last report card from school. All comparisons are significant at $p < .001$. Time Mgmt, Self-Management to Time subscale; Self-Organization, Self-Organization/Problem Solving subscale; Emotion Regulation, Self-Regulation of Emotion subscale.

students: *M*, 106.9, *SD* = 34.2; C–F students: *M*, 149.6, *SD* = 51.3 (F = 292.45, p < .001). These analyses provide yet further evidence for the validity of the BDEFS-CA in showing that parental reports of EF deficits on the scale are significantly associated with a child's school grades.

School Adjustment

Information was also available from parents on whether or not their children's teachers had told the parents during the past year that their children were having significant problems with their behavior or school performance. A comparison of the 501 children receiving such reports with the 1,409 children who did not receive them shows that the former are having significantly more problems with EF deficits in daily life on the BDEFS-CA. The results of these comparisons are also shown in Table 8.7 for all 10 BDEFS-CA scores. Parents were also asked whether their children had ever been retained in a grade. There were 102 children who had been so retained, and they were compared with the remainder (N = 1,812) on the BDEFS-CA subscale scores. All comparisons were significant at p < .001, and the results for the five subscale domain scores are shown in Figure 8.7. Here one can see that children who had been retained had significantly more EF deficits across all five subscales than did those who had never been retained in a grade in school. The mean scores for the EF Summary Score were also significantly elevated in the group that had been retained: retained: M = 140.7, SD = 54.8; not retained: M = 111.8, SD = 38.6 (F = 51.15, p < .001). Results for the other BDEFS-CA scores were comparable to these and significant at p < .001. As another index of school adjustment, parents reported whether their child had ever been suspended or expelled from school.

TABLE 8.7. BDEFS-CA Long and Short Form Scores for Children Who Received Teacher Reports of Significant Behavior or School Performance Problems at School during the Past Year and Those Who Received No Such Teacher Reports

	No problems (N = 1,409)		School problems (N = 501)			
Subscale	Mean	*SD*	Mean	*SD*	*F*	*p*
Self-Management to Time	21.1	6.9	30.7	9.6	564.15	< .001
Self-Organization	17.8	5.3	24.7	10.1	378.33	< .001
Self-Restraint	18.9	6.0	28.0	10.4	562.38	< .001
Self-Motivation	20.2	6.9	31.6	11.1	717.92	< .001
Self-Reg. of Emotion	22.8	8.1	33.5	13.3	452.33	< .001
Total EF Summary Score	100.8	28.1	148.6	47.4	722.76	< .001
ADHD-EF Index	13.8	3.8	20.1	6.6	665.36	< .001
EF Symptom Count	4.5	8.8	21.5	20.5	637.73	< .001
EF Summary Score—Short Form	29.6	8.3	43.3	13.7	686.59	< .001
EF Symptom Count—Short Form	1.5	2.7	6.5	6.0	605.94	< .001

Note. F, results for the *F*-test; *p*, probability value for the *F*-test if ≤ .05; Self-Organization, Self-Organization/Problem Solving subscale; Self-Reg. of Emotion, Self-Regulation of Emotion subscale.

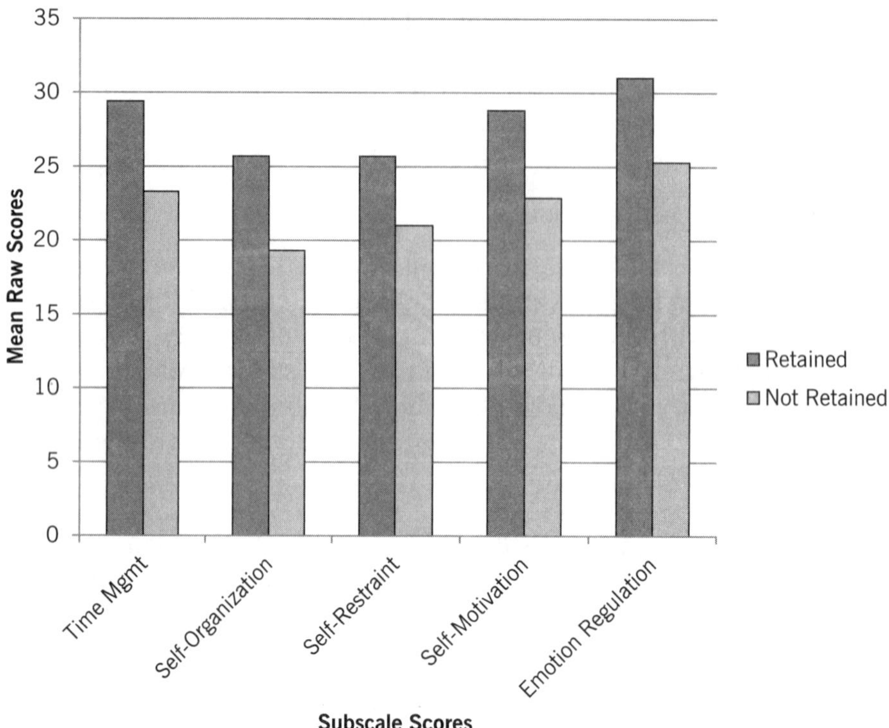

FIGURE 8.7. Mean raw scores for the five BDEFS-CA subscales for children who were reported by parents to have ever been retained a grade in school to those not having been retained. All comparisons are significant at $p < .001$. Time Mgmt, Self-Management to Time subscale; Self-Organization, Self-Organization/Problem Solving subscale; Emotion Regulation, Self-Regulation of Emotion subscale.

The comparison of these two groups to each other is shown in Table 8.8. Obviously, these results make it clear that children experiencing suspension or expulsion have higher EF deficit scores on all BDEFS-CA scores than do those who never had this experience. All of this evidence indicates that EF deficits as rated on the BDEFS-CA are significantly related to various indices of school adjustment (behavior or performance problems, grade retention, and suspensions or expulsions). Here again we find substantial evidence for the validity of the BDEFS-CA scores and for the importance of EF to school adjustment.

Accidental Injuries and Poisonings

Children with psychiatric disorders are known to be at increased risk for accidental injuries (Rowe, Maughan, & Goodman, 2004). After controlling for comorbidity with other disorders and some psychosocial risk factors, research shows that ODD may be more associated with burns and poisonings, whereas ADHD is linked to risk for fractures (Rowe et al., 2004). Depression and anxiety may also be linked to certain injury types as well. Children with ADHD in particular have been shown to be at a significantly increased risk for accidental injuries and poisonings (Barkley, 2006;

TABLE 8.8. BDEFS-CA Long and Short Form Scores for Children Who Had or Had Not Been Suspended/Expelled from School

	Not suspended (*N* = 1,783)		Suspended/ expelled (*N* = 129)			
Subscale	Mean	*SD*	Mean	*SD*	*F*	*p*
Self-Management to Time	23.1	8.4	31.3	11.1	109.36	< .001
Self-Organization	19.2	7.2	24.8	9.5	67.31	< .001
Self-Restraint	20.6	7.8	30.1	11.5	163.59	< .001
Self-Motivation	22.5	9.1	32.5	11.8	140.44	< .001
Self-Reg. of Emotion	24.9	10.1	35.2	14.8	116.50	< .001
Total EF Summary Score	110.4	37.5	154.0	52.1	152.40	< .001
ADHD-EF Index	15.1	5.2	20.5	7.0	123.24	< .001
EF Symptom Count	7.8	13.6	24.4	21.9	160.51	< .001
EF Summary Score—Short Form	32.4	10.9	45.1	14.9	154.40	< .001
EF Symptom Count—Short Form	2.5	4.1	7.4	6.4	158.21	< .001

Note. F, results for the *F*-test; *p*, probability value for the *F*-test if ≤ .05; Self-Organization, Self-Organization/Problem Solving subscale; Self-Reg. of Emotion, Self-Regulation of Emotion subscale.

Hinshaw, 2002). Given that all psychiatric disorders were found to be linked to EF deficits (see Chapter 7) and that such deficits are especially prominent in ADHD, it is possible that EF deficits are therefore related to risk for accidental injuries or poisonings. We asked parents to report on how many times their children had to be taken to a doctor or hospital for treatment of an accidental injury or poisoning. The majority of children (*N* = 1,309; 69%) had never had such an event, whereas 18% had just one such event, and 5% had experienced three or more such events. This latter group was therefore considered to be injury prone. They were compared on the BDEFS-CA subscales with those having two or fewer such injuries or poisonings. The results are shown in Table 8.9, and all comparisons were significant, although the mean differences were small. This indicates, nevertheless, that children who are accident prone are more likely to have EF deficits on the BDEFS-CA than those who are not so prone, once again providing evidence for the validity of the BDEFS-CA. The reverse comparisons were also done to determine whether children deficient in each of the five EF domains on the long form (≥ 93rd percentile) were more likely to be accident prone. Results indicated that those deficient in four of the five subscale domains were more likely to be prone to accidental injuries. For instance, those deficient in Self-Management to Time were almost twice as likely to be accident prone than those not so deficient (8.4 vs. 4.5%; $\chi^2 = 5.31$, $p = .02$). This was also true for those deficient in Self-Restraint (8.8 vs. 4.5%; $\chi^2 = 6.75$, $p = .009$). The risk was slightly greater for those deficient in the Self-Motivation (10.1 vs. 4.3%; $\chi^2 = 12.26$, $p < .001$) and Self-Regulation of Emotion domains (10.3 vs. 4.3%; $\chi^2 = 12.12$, $p < .001$). Overall, those deficient in the overall EF Summary Score were twice as likely to be prone to accidental injuries (8.8 vs. 4.5%; $\chi^2 = 6.12$, $p = .013$). Thus there is a small but significant link between certain EF deficits on the BDEFS-CA and risk for accidental injuries. Here again is evidence of the validity of the BDEFS-CA.

TABLE 8.9. BDEFS-CA Long and Short Form Scores for Children Who Had Three or More Accidental Injuries or Poisonings (Accident Prone) and Those Having Two or Fewer

	Not accident prone (N= 1,812)		Accident prone (N= 93)			
Subscale	Mean	*SD*	Mean	*SD*	*F*	*p*
Self-Management to Time	23.5	8.7	27.0	10.2	14.03	< .001
Self-Organization	19.5	7.4	21.6	9.6	7.08	.008
Self-Restraint	21.1	8.3	24.9	10.4	18.34	< .001
Self-Motivation	23.0	9.4	26.9	11.9	14.19	< .001
Self-Reg. of Emotion	25.4	10.5	30.0	14.2	16.45	< .001
Total EF Summary Score	112.6	39.3	130.5	51.1	17.79	< .001
ADHD-EF Index	15.3	5.4	17.6	7.0	15.12	< .001
EF Symptom Count	8.7	14.6	14.9	19.8	15.74	< .001
EF Summary Score—Short Form	33.0	11.4	38.2	14.6	18.05	< .001
EF Symptom Count—Short Form	2.7	4.3	4.7	5.7	17.00	< .001

Note. F, results for the *F*-test; *p*, probability value for the *F*-test if ≤ .05; Self-Organization, Self-Organization/Problem Solving subscale; Self-Reg. of Emotion, Self-Regulation of Emotion subscale.

Conclusion

The findings presented in this and the previous chapter provide varied and substantial evidence for the construct, convergent, divergent, criterion, and ecological validity of the BDEFS-CA scores. Differing patterns of subscale scores were evident across various neurological, developmental, learning, and psychiatric disorders (see Chapter 7). The scores were also significantly associated with various forms of psychiatric, psychological, and educational treatments in the sense that children placing in the clinically deficient range of the BDEFS-CA were significantly more likely to be receiving such services. It is also clear that BDEFS-CA scores are related to impairment in major life activities in each of the 15 domains of the BFIS-CA. Children having greater EF deficits are more likely to be rated by parents as being more impaired across all of these domains. This linkage of BDEFS-CA scores to impairment was also found in analyses of more specific areas of psychosocial impairment, such as community activities and sports participation, friendships and unpopularity, school adjustment (grades, retentions, suspensions and expulsions), and proneness to accidental injuries or poisonings. Higher scores on the BDEFS-CA were associated with greater risks across all of these domains to varying yet significant degrees. Such findings make the BDEFS-CA among the most validated parent rating scales of EF deficits in children currently available. All of these areas are clearly in need of more research, but what research exists supports the validity of the scale. Currently lacking research is the sensitivity of the BDEFS-CA scores to various treatments recommended for the management of EF deficits. But the available evidence concerning validity supports the use of the BDEFS-CA in various clinical, scientific, educational, and other organizational settings in which the assessment of children's EF deficits in daily life is of interest.

CHAPTER 9

Scoring and Interpretation of the BDEFS-CA Forms

As with the adult version of the BDEFS (Barkley, 2011a), the BDEFS-CA can be used to evaluate EF in the daily life activities of children ages 6–17 years quickly and inexpensively in a clinical practice, research setting, or educational or organizational setting, among others. The BDEFS-CA is intended to be used by trained professionals in clinical, research, or educational/organizational specialties who have sufficient educational background and experience in the evaluation of child psychological functioning and its impairment. Interpretation of the BDEFS-CA scales, scores, and profiles requires graduate training in a psychological, psychiatric, educational, or medical specialty which provides relevant training and coursework in the administration and interpretation of psychological measures in an accredited college or university. Besides carefully reviewing and understanding this manual, examiners using the BDEFS-CA should be familiar with the *Standards for Educational and Psychological Testing* of the American Psychological Association (1999).

BDEFS-CA Materials

The original long form of the BDEFS-CA (70 items) is likely to yield more reliable information because of the greater length of the subscales and hence the total scale. But where time is of the essence, the 20-item BDEFS-CA Short Form can be used as a quick screen for the likelihood that a child or adolescent is experiencing EF deficits in his/her daily life activities. Where clinically significant problems are evident, then a follow-up evaluation can be done with the long form if the examiner wishes to obtain broader coverage of the specific domains of EF in daily life activities. Only the long form version of the BDEFS-CA yields subscale scores for the five major dimensions of EF problems in daily life activities identified in Chapters 4 and 5: Self-Management to Time, Self-Organization/Problem Solving, Self-Restraint, Self-Motivation, and Self-Regulation of Emotion. Because the short form contains only 20 items, separate scores for each domain are not provided nor recommended; only 4 items sample each domain, and this number is not believed to be sufficient to render a confident evaluation of that domain. A Total EF Summary Score is computed for both the long and short form versions of the BDEFS-CA based on the entire scale's content. And a 10-item ADHD-EF Index can be scored from the long form if the risk for ADHD in the child or adolescent is of interest in the examination. Finally, the examiner can compute an EF Symptom Count score for each version of the scale; this may be especially informative in clinical settings. A clinically significant symptom of an EF deficit is defined here as any item answered as occurring "often" (3) or "very often" (4). This threshold for defining an item as an EF symptom is based on the responses of the normative sample that indicated that such answers were uncommon in that sample (see Table 4.2).

The BDEFS-CA Long Form can be scored using one of four EF Profiles, depending on the child's age group (6–11, 12–17) and sex. The BDEFS-CA Short Form is also provided in the Appendix. Only a single EF Profile is provided for the short form in the Appendix because only the EF Summary Score and EF Symptom Count are computed from that version. Those scores are then recorded on the EF Profile for the short form in the appropriate columns for the child's age group and sex.

Appropriate Purposes and Populations for the BDEFS-CA

The BDEFS-CA forms are not intended to replicate or replace the use of neuropsychological tests of EF. Indeed, the two types of measures are only modestly related if at all, and so neither can replace the other nor serve as an alternative means of measuring the same EF components (see Chapter 1). Instead, EF is best viewed as a hierarchically organized series of levels or outwardly projecting concentric rings of the extended phenotype of EF into humans' major life activities (Barkley, 2012b). EF tests and EF ratings are likely evaluating quite different levels of this extended phenotype of EF, much the way lab measures of reaction time and a parent rating scale of a teen's safe driving habits while operating a motor vehicle are measuring very different levels of driving performance. In the former case, they are mostly assessing cold cognition at the initial *Instrumental–Self-Directed* level of EF, perhaps at its most proximal juncture with activity in the PFC and its networks to other brain regions; hence the focus on these tests and other lab measures as possible endophenotypes for EF (or ADHD). Even then, they are limited by their focus on cold cognition, absence of emotional self-regulation, dearth of social goals or purposes, limited ascertainment window, and clinic context, among other problems noted in Chapter 1. EF ratings, in contrast, are likely assessing EF at its *Methodical–Self-reliant* and *Tactical–Reciprocal* levels that occur in daily life activities and social relations. Other measures, such as adaptive behavior inventories, social skills rating scales, and even measures of moral conduct in social settings are needed to tap the *Strategic–Cooperative* and eventual *Principled–Mutualistic* level attained by adulthood, as described in my recent text (Barkley, 2012b). Measures of impairment, such as archival records (school report cards, achievement tests, transcripts) and rating scales of functional effectiveness in major domains of children's life activities, such as the BFIS-CA (Barkley, 2012a), are also needed to assess the consequences associated with deficient EF in daily life. Therefore, the selection of a measure or set of measures of EF should be based largely on the purposes of the evaluation and the levels of EF one wishes to assess. If evaluating the lowest, instrumental, moment-to-moment level of cold cognitive functioning believed to represent basic EF components is of importance, then EF tests or batteries might be preferred to EF ratings in daily life. This may be the case in neuroimaging research, molecular genetics of the instrumental EFs, or in the brain localization of specific EF functions, for which the EF tests and batteries may be useful. The point is arguable given the numerous problems evident in using tests to measure EF, discussed in Chapter 1. If, however, the purpose of the evaluation is to identify EF at higher levels of greater behavioral complexity over longer terms and in socially significant settings and domains of daily life activities and to predict the likelihood of impairment in various domains of major life activities, then the BDEFS-CA would be of greater utility than would EF tests.

The BDEFS-CA is intended to be used for the evaluation of individuals between 6 and 17 years of age. From age 18 to age 81, the adult BDEFS (Barkley, 2011a) can be used to evaluate EF in daily life activities. Typically, the children being evaluated will be those who reside in the United States, as this country is the source for the normative sample. Use of the BDEFS-CA with populations, countries, cultures, or ethnic groups outside of the United States may be inappropriate to the extent that such groups may vary from the normative reference sample described in this manual.

Administration

The BDEFS-CA Long Form or Short Form should be given directly to the parent whose child is being evaluated for completion, along with a clear explanation of the purposes for which the ratings are being obtained. The examiner should also clearly explain the instructions for completing the rating scale (see the BDEFS-CA scales in the Appendix), and the parent should have the opportunity to raise concerns or questions about the scale. The BDEFS-CA may be mailed out to parents to complete before the day of the intended evaluation. In this case the scale should be accompanied by a cover letter that explains how the scale will be used and the instructions for its completion. This letter should also give the parent a means of contacting the examiner regarding any concerns or questions he/she might have about the scale or its intended purpose.

The BDEFS-CA Long Form takes an average of approximately 10–15 minutes to complete by the average parent in the general population, whereas the BDEFS-CA Short Form may take only about 3–5 minutes to complete. If the parent is completing the form in person, the examiner should review the scale for any missed items, then encourage the rater to complete those items. The failure to complete more than a few items on the scale is likely to invalidate the resulting scores and make the use of the normative tables on the EF Profiles inappropriate. If the scale was returned by mail and items were missing, have the parent complete them on the day of the evaluation. If there is simply no further opportunity to get any missed items completed, then these items should be answered with a 1 (*never* or *rarely*) to create a conservative bias to the scores such that EF deficits are not unduly exaggerated. Even then, the failure to complete more than 5% of the items on the scale should be considered sufficient cause to invalidate the scale (4+ items on the full BDEFS-CA Long Form, 2+ items on the BDEFS-CA Short Form).

Scoring and Interpreting the BDEFS-CA Long Form (70 Items)

Follow these procedures to score the BDEFS-CA Long Form:

- The easiest method for scoring is to start with Section 1 (Self-Management to Time items). Add all of the answers circled in this section to get the total raw score. Write the answer in the line marked Section 1 Total Score in the shaded row at the end of this section. If you prefer, you can do this by an alternate means. Add all of the answers that are circled "1" (*Never or rarely*) in Column 2 of this section (the actual items are in Column 1). Place that sum in the empty box below that column (the box is in the shaded row marked "Office Use Only"). Now do the same for Column 3—sum all of the circled answers of "2's" (*Sometimes*) in this column and place that sum at the bottom of that column in the empty box. Repeat this process for columns 4 (circled answers of *Often*, or 3's) and 5 (*Very Often*, or 4's). Now add these four sums together to get the total score for Section 1. Write the answer in the line marked Section 1 Total Score. Again, this will be in the shaded row at the end of this section. This takes less than 15 or 20 seconds to do per section.

- Repeat this same procedure for Sections 2–5 to get the total score for each of those sections. These section scores correspond to each of the five subscales of the BDEFS-CA Long Form: Section 1, Self-Management to Time; Section 2, Self-Organization/Problem Solving; Section 3, Self-Restraint; Section 4, Self-Motivation; and Section 5, Self-Regulation of Emotion.

- When you have computed each of these section total scores, add them up to get the EF Summary Score, which is the total score for all items on the entire scale. Place the answer in the line at the end of the scale marked "EF Summary Score" (this line is also shaded and marked "Office Use Only").

- Finally, go back over the entire scale and count the number of items that were answered with a 3 (*Often*) or a 4 (*Very Often*) to get the EF Symptom Count. Enter this number in the box so labeled in the last line of the scale, again marked "For Office Use Only."

You have now computed seven scores for the BDEFS-CA Long Form—the five subscale total raw scores, the EF Summary Score (sum of the five subscale scores), and the EF Symptom Count. If you wish, you can compute an eighth score: the ADHD-EF Index.

ADHD-EF Index

If you wish to compute the ADHD-EF Index to evaluate the likelihood that the child or adolescent may have ADHD, then add up the scores on the form for the 10 items that constitute this index. Place that sum in the last line of the scale where you see the ADHD-EF Index score indicated in the shaded row marked "Office Use Only." The 10 items that make up this index are: **5, 20, 21, 23, 27, 35, 47, 51, 59,** and **68**. They are indicated on the scale with **boldfaced** and underscored item number. These items are also listed in the last line of the scale in the shaded line.

As a general rule, the following scores or higher ones for each age group and sex on the ADHD-EF Index are reasonable to use to identify children as at risk for ADHD: males ages 6–11 years = 26; males ages 12–17 years = 27; females ages 6–11 years = 23; and females ages 12–17 years = 24. These scores represent the 93rd percentile for these age groups and sex, which is approximately +1.5 *SD*'s above the mean for the general population. *This Index is not the sole basis for nor a substitute for a clinical evaluation and eventual diagnosis of ADHD in a child or adolescent—it is just an indicator of risk for ADHD.* Anyone scoring at or above these levels should be considered a candidate for a more thorough clinical evaluation in order to determine the presence of a diagnosis of ADHD and any need for treatment of it.

Using the BDEFS-CA EF Profiles

- Select the BDEFS-CA EF Profile form (see the Appendix) suitable for the child's sex and age group (6–11 or 12–17). Up to eight scores are possible from the long form: five subscale domain scores, EF Summary Score, EF Symptom Count, and ADHD-EF Index.

- Write the raw score you computed for each of these eight types of scores in the cells in the bottom row of that profile—place the score in the column with the heading of the name of that scale (e.g., Self-Management to Time). Each column of this profile shows a range of potential raw scores for each of the eight scores computed from the long form.

- Starting at the left-hand column of the table, under Self-Management to Time, circle the score (or score range) in this column that reflects the respondent's raw score for Section 1 of the BDEFS-CA Long Form. Look to the far left column to determine the percentile of the general population that this score represents.

- The higher the percentile, the more deviant is the score relative to the normative sample (general population). The percentiles that reflect the typical range of deficits are shown as ranges (1–9, 10–19, 20–29, 30–39, 40–49, 50–59, 60–69 and then as individual percentiles starting at 70 and up to 99+. Raw scores are collapsed into ranges of scores at the lower percentiles for two reasons: (1) a large number of scores in the general population are found here, making the correspondence of each score to a single percentile difficult if not impossible; and (2) scores in these lower percentile ranges generally have little clinical significance other than to indicate that this individual is not elevated or abnormal in his/her level of EF deficits in that domain of EF. However, scores in the highest quartile begin to take on some clinical significance as indicators of clinical deficiency and risks for impairments. For that reason, individual percentiles are provided for each raw score above the 70th percentile threshold.

• Generally, scores from the 76th to 84th percentiles should be considered of *marginal* clinical significance. Those between the 85th and 92nd percentiles would be considered *borderline* or *somewhat deficient.* Those between the 93rd and 95th percentiles would be *mildly deficient.* Those between the 96th and 98th percentiles would be considered *moderately deficient.* And those at the 99th percentile would be viewed as *markedly deficient* or *severe.*

• Now do the same for the Self-Organization/Problem Solving raw score (the total raw score from Section 2 of the Self-Report scale)—that is, circle the score in this column that represents the raw score for Section 2 of the long form rating scale. Look to either the far left or far right column to see the percentile score associated with this raw score.

• Repeat this procedure for the raw scores from Sections 3–5 (Self-Restraint, Self-Motivation, and Self-Regulation of Emotion).

• Then follow the same procedure to get the percentile for the EF Summary Score, EF Symptom Count, and ADHD-EF Index using their respective columns of the EF profile.

• To create a more visually obvious profile, you can draw lines that connect the circles you made around each raw score in each column. Start at the far left side for Self-Management to Time and draw a line connecting the circle in this column to the one in the next column (Self-Organization/Problem Solving) and so on until you have lines connecting all the circles from left to right across the profile.

• In general, the higher the percentile represented by that child's score, the greater is the likelihood that the individual is deficient in that domain of EF and that he/she may experience some impairment in major life activities as a consequence of his/her increasing level of EF deficits in daily life activities.

Scoring the BDEFS-CA Short Form (20 Items)

The scoring of the BDEFS-CA Short Form is obviously easier given that only 20 items need to be considered for scoring compared with the 70-item Long Form.

• First, sum the answers circled in Column 2 (answer of "1" or *Never or rarely*) and enter this at the bottom of that column in the shaded area. Do the same for columns 3, 4, and 5 (values of 2, 3, and 4), entering these sums in the empty cell at the bottom of their respective columns. Now add these raw scores together to get the total EF Summary Score for the short form.

• Separate scores are not computed for subscales, such as Self-Management to Time or Self-Motivation, as was done on the long form. Again, the reason is that only four items come from each of those subscales, and that is not enough of a sample to be considered a reliable indicator of that EF domain. The short form is used simply to get a quick assessment of possible deficits in EF generally considered.

• Finally, review the scale responses and count the number of items that were answered with a 3 (*Often*) or a 4 (*Very often*). This is the EF Symptom Count. Enter this where indicated on the last line of the scale.

• Use the BDEFS-CA Short Form EF Profile page to convert raw scores to percentiles. This sheet contains a single table to be used for both sexes and both age groups. In the table you will find two columns for each of the two age groups and each sex. The first column under each age group and sex is for the EF Summary Score, and the second column is for the EF Symptom Count. These are the only two scores for which norms are provided for this short form.

• Write the child's two raw scores that you computed from the short form into the appropriate cell on the bottom line of this EF Profile under the appropriate columns for his/her age group and sex.

• Then look up the first of those two columns for the score or range of scores that corresponds to this child's EF Summary Score. Circle this score. Look either to the left or right far column to locate the percentile (or percentile range) that corresponds to that score.

• Then circle the raw score for the EF Symptom Count in the column to the right that is for this same age group. Once more, look to the far left or far right columns to find the percentile that corresponds to this score relative to the general population for that age group.

BDEFS-CA Interview

Very rarely, situations may arise in which an individual being evaluated is unable to complete the BDEFS-CA Long Form or BDEFS-CA Short Form, perhaps because they cannot read, cannot read English, or have a sufficiently severe visual impairment that precludes completing these rating scales. In these instances, the examiner may opt to use the BDEFS-CA Interview, which is based on the BDEFS-CA Short Form (20 items). Examiners are strongly encouraged to use the BDEFS-CA rating scales whenever possible, as there are no norms that are directly applicable to the interview form. But in these rare circumstances, the examiner can conduct a short interview using this Interview Form to see whether the individual has significant deficits in EF in daily life activities.

Instructions to be read to the person being interviewed are provided at the top of the interview form. The individual is to be asked whether his/her child has experienced each item during the past 6 months to a degree that is *often or more frequent* relative to other individuals of his/her age group. The examiner simply places a check in either the Yes or No columns based on the response of the participant to each question. After the interview, add up the number of Yes responses to get the EF Symptom Count. Although no norms are available for this interview form, it has been found to be highly correlated with the BDEFS-CA rating scale. Therefore, to gain a very rough estimate of how deviant the parent-reports about a child may be, simply look at the norms on the EF Profile for the BDEFS-CA Short Form. Find the columns for that child's age group and sex. Look under the specific column for the EF Symptom Count for that person's age group and sex. Find his/her raw score in the EF Symptom Count column for the appropriate age group and sex and circle it. Then look at the far left or far right column to see the percentile that corresponds to this raw score. Examiners must understand that this provides only a very rough approximation of the status of this individual relative to others in the population using this table as the interview form was not given to people in the normative sample. This is the reason that examiners are encouraged to use the rating scale versions of the BDEFS-CA forms whenever possible.

Using the BDEFS-CA to Evaluate Response to Treatment

Both of the BDEFS-CA Forms can be valuable tools in evaluating an individual's response to treatment, such as cognitive training as part of neurorehabilitation interventions, cognitive-behavioral treatment, or medication treatments, for example, the use of ADHD medications. Although the BDEFS-CA Long Form can be used for this purpose, the Short Form provides a less time-consuming and more cost-effective means of doing so.

How much change in a score would be needed to interpret that change as reliable? That is, how much change can be viewed as likely being the result of the intervention? Scientists and clinicians have employed various methods to determine how much change should be considered as a positive (or negative) response to treatment—for instance, a change of 20, 30, or 40% from the baseline score. These, however, are quite arbitrary thresholds. Instead, several statistical approaches exist that are better for this purpose. Unlike such arbitrarily defined thresholds for change, these statistical approaches take into consideration the test–retest reliability of the measure and the variation in change scores in the general population. Of these various approaches, one used quite frequently is the reliable change index (RCI) developed by Jacobson and colleagues (Jacobson, Roberts, Berns, & McGlinchey, 1999; Jacobson & Truax, 1991). This approach ensures that the degree of change exceeds that which may result merely from measurement error or unreliability. In essence, it shows whether the change in the scores from pre- to posttreatment can be assumed, with 95% confidence (probability), to have come from a different distribution than that occurring as a consequence of variation and unreliability alone. A difference in scores of a magnitude at or exceeding the RCI number (threshold) would be expected less than 5% of the time by chance and unreliability of measurement alone.

The formula for calculating an RCI is $X_2 - X_1/S_{diff}$, where X_2 is the individual's posttest score and X_1 is his/her pretest score. The difference between the two is then divided by the standard error of the difference scores (S_{diff}). S_{diff} can be obtained directly from our results by using the standard deviations, as well as the test–retest reliability information for each scale, inserted into the formula provided in the article by Jacobson and Truax (1991). The difference in means is divided by the S_{diff}. Where the resultant number equals or exceeds 1.96, the difference is considered reliable (to occur 5% or less of the time by chance alone).

To save you time, the values of RCI needed to be considered a significant change on each subscale of the BDEFS-CA have been calculated. Those values for RCI for the long and short forms of the BDEFS-CA are shown in Table 9.1 for each age group and sex. To use them, simply take the posttest score of a patient or participant and subtract it from his/her pretest score. Then look in Table 9.1 in the row that corresponds to the subscale being used to evaluate change. Look in the column of that row for the patient's age group and sex. If this difference in the patient's scores meets or exceeds the score in this cell of the table, then the change in pre- to posttest scores can be considered to be reliable, or outside the range of error of the measure. Probably the best score to use in these cases would be the EF Summary Score, but the subscale scores of the BDEFS-CA Long Form can also be examined for their reliable change if that is of interest. If the BDEFS-CA Short Form is being used for this purpose, then it is recommended that one use only the EF Summary Score.

The fact that a change in scores is reliable does not necessarily make it clinically significant or meaningful. One means of determining such significance is to determine whether the child now falls within the normal range following the intervention. That is, does the child's score after treatment allow one to conclude that it likely came from the normal range of scores in the general population? For this determination, Jacobson and Truax (1991) recommended that the posttreatment score now place within 2 *SD*'s of the mean, or below the 98th percentile, for the normal population. This is a fairly generous interpretation of normalization. Others, such as myself, recommend that the posttreatment score place within 1.5 *SD*'s of the normal mean, or approximately the 93rd percentile, as this is a threshold often used to determine whether someone is clinically symptomatic or not. These demarcations for the general population sample for each age group are provided in Table 9.2. Thus if a patient, following treatment, has shown (1) a change in scores from pre-testing to posttesting that meets or surpasses the RCI score in Table 9.1 *and* (2) a final posttest score within +1.5 *SD*'s or +2 *SD*'s of the mean for the normative sample (depending on how lenient the definition of recovery is chosen to be), one could conclude that the treatment had resulted not only in reliable change but also in recovery or normalization.

TABLE 9.1. The RCI Necessary for Pre- to Posttreatment Difference Scores to Be Significant (Reliable) on the BDEFS-CA Long Form Subscales and the Short Form EF Summary Score

	RCI by age group and sex			
	6–11 years		12–17 years	
Subscale	Males	Females	Males	Females
Self-Management to Time	12.7	11.5	13.8	12.4
Self-Organization/Problem Solving	10.1	9.3	11.3	9.3
Self-Restraint	11.7	10.5	11.9	10.6
Self-Motivation	12.5	11.4	14.0	11.7
Self-Regulation of Emotion	13.3	12.8	12.7	12.1
EF Summary Score	48.3	44.4	51.4	44.6
EF Summary Score—Short Form	14.8	13.8	16.1	14.2

TABLE 9.2. Thresholds for Determining Normalization or Recovery at Posttesting after Treatment

	Age group and sex							
	6–11 Years				12–17 Years			
	Males		Females		Males		Females	
Subscale	+1.5	+2.0	+1.5	+2.0	+1.5	+2.0	+1.5	+2.0
Self-Management to Time	37	41	34	38	40	45	36	40
Self-Organization/Problem Solving	31	35	29	33	33	37	30	33
Self-Restraint	36	40	32	36	35	40	32	36
Self-Motivation	38	43	35	39	41	47	36	40
Self-Regulation of Emotion	44	49	42	47	41	47	40	45
EF Summary Score	179	200	165	184	183	205	166	185
EF Summary Score—Short Form	51	57	48	53	54	60	49	55

Note. Thresholds are provided for +1.5 and +2 *SD*'s above the mean of the normative sample for each age group for the BDEFS-CA Long Form subscales and the Short Form EF Summary Score.

As an example, consider a male child within the age range of 6–11 years with ADHD or even a closed head injury who is manifesting significant deficits in EF in daily life as reflected in an EF Summary Score from the BDEFS-CA Long Form of 260. According to the table of norms in the EF Profile for a boy of this age for the long form, this patient is above the 99th percentile of the population of his age group and sex. Following the introduction of treatment for a month with an ADHD medication, the parent of this child completes the BDEFS-CA Long Form again; the child now has an EF Summary Score of 160. Is this degree of change from the medication treatment reliable? That is, is it likely to fall outside the realm of merely measurement error or unreliability? To find out, compute the RCI as follows: pretest score (260) minus posttest score (160) = 100 points. Table 9.1 shows that for 6- to 11-year-old boys the RCI needed to be significant, for the EF Summary Score is 48.3. The patient's change score of 100 is well above this RCI threshold. Thus the clinician can feel confident that the improvement in EF deficits is not simply due to measurement error or unreliability. It is likely a consequence of the treatment. It is reliable. The patient could be considered a treatment responder in this instance (assuming that side effects of the medication are not so annoying as to warrant treatment discontinuation).

Next we wish to know whether the child has been normalized by the treatment—that is, whether the intervention has brought him to within the normal range. Examine Table 9.2 to see the threshold EF Summary Score for +2 *SD*'s above the normal mean for boys ages 6–11 years. The Summary Score is 200, which corresponds to approximately the 98th percentile. The patient's posttest score of 160 is well below this figure, and so it could be considered within the broadly defined normal range. However, as noted earlier, some clinicians and researchers believe that this is too generous a definition of normalcy for determining recovery. Using the criterion of +1.5 *SD*'s above the normal mean may be preferred. In that case, see the appropriate column in Table 9.2, where we find that this threshold is 179. The patient's posttest score of 160 is also below this level. And so even by this more conservative definition of normalization, the patient can be considered to place within the broadly defined normal range for his age group and sex following treatment. This may be considered "recovery." In fact, according to the norms on the Long Form EF Profile for males ages 6–11, this patient's score is at the 86th percentile for the general population. By this empirical approach to defining a treatment responder (RCI) and normalization, the treatment has been successful.

Of course, ADHD medications provide only symptomatic relief in such cases, and only when the medication is taken at therapeutic levels. Therefore, the resulting reliable change (positive response) and normalization refer only to a temporary effect of the medication while in use and not to a permanent alteration of the patient's functioning in the absence of medication management. Although the BDEFS-CA Long Form was used in this example, it would be more efficient (less time-consuming and more economical) in this case to have used the BDEFS-CA Short Form and the EF Summary Score from that considerably shorter scale.

To add further to the utility of such an evaluation of an ADHD medication, a clinician might want to have the parent complete the Side Effects Questionnaire (Barkley & Murphy, 2006) both before and after treatment to ensure that the changes taking place in any reported adverse events are in fact a consequence of the medication and not merely preexisting conditions that went unexamined prior to the medication trial.

Evaluating Change in EF Due to Brain Injury

A very similar approach can be taken to evaluating whether or not a child or teen has experienced a significant deterioration in his/her EF in daily life activities following some form of brain injury, whether the origin is from a traumatic, infectious, cancerous, or vascular event or other causal factor. The clinician here may be asking the question, Has a reliable and significant decline in EF in daily life occurred in this patient? The RCI figures in Table 9.1 can be used to determine whether the deterioration in functioning is reliable (probably outside the realm of measurement error). The parent can complete the BDEFS-CA on how he/she believes his/her child is functioning now. He/she can then complete a second version with reference to how well he/she believes the child was functioning prior to the event. Then the clinician can compare the patient's premorbid and postmorbid EF Summary Scores.

Once again, to get the RCI, subtract the postmorbid from the premorbid score, which in this case will be negative. Now look in Table 9.1 for the EF Summary Score for the patient's age group and sex. If the difference in the patient's scores is higher than the one in the table, the patient's deterioration in functioning can be considered to be reliable—that is, the change is probably outside the realm of measurement error or unreliability (likely to occur 5% or less of the time). The thresholds provided in Table 9.2 for age group and this BDEFS-CA score can now be used to determine whether this patient's scores now places him/her outside of the normal range using both the +1.5 *SD*'s and +2 *SD*'s thresholds (approximately the 93rd and 98th percentiles). That is to say that the patient's postmorbid score is now more likely to have been drawn from a distribution of individuals impaired or disordered in their EF in daily life activities than to have been drawn from the general adult population.

Evaluating Change in EF Due to Psychiatric Disorders or Emotionally Traumatic Events

As I explained in the manual for the adult BDEFS (Barkley, 2011a), events that lead to changes in EF in daily life activities, even those that may be relatively transient, do not always have to originate in some injury to the brain and especially the PFC. The conflating of EF with PFC functioning and hence of these two distinct yet partially coupled levels of analysis (neuropsychological vs. neurological) can mislead clinicians and others into believing that only injuries to the brain can result in deficits in EF in daily life activities. It is just as possible that psychiatric disorders having a developmental origin, such as ADHD, learning disorders, or autism, and likely arising from genetically and even environmentally influenced subtle maldevelopment of the brain (as in risk gene × toxin interactions in ADHD) can give rise to deficits in EF in daily life activities. Indeed, as shown in earlier chapters, ADHD, regardless of its etiology, is highly likely to be associated with such deficits in daily life activities, even if it is less evident on neuropsychological tests of EF. As noted in Chapter 1, this disparity in the results from EF ratings versus EF tests has been found to be the case for various neurodevelopmental disorders besides ADHD. In short, the absence of evidence of brain injury in cases manifesting significant deficits in EF in daily life activities as measured by scales such as the BDEFS-CA does not in any way preclude the possibility that such deficits exist and are legitimate. Evidence of neurological etiology is not a prerequisite for establishing the validity of deficits in EF in daily life activities.

It is also possible for individuals even with typical brain development to experience episodic deficits in EF in daily life activities as a consequence of psychiatric disorders that are not always developmental in origin, such as depression and anxiety. Such disorders of mood may be sufficiently profound to interfere with the adequate or effective utilization of EF, especially in daily life activities, even if the neurological system underlying EF is itself uncompromised. The ubiquitous feedback loops and networks known to exist in brain functioning and especially in the relationship of the PFC to numerous other non-EF systems make it very possible for disorders that do not originate in the EF system (or PFC for that matter) to nonetheless have a detrimental effect on the execution of EF in daily life activities. Just as not all brain disorders lead to disruption of the EF system or its effective use in daily life activities, so all disruptions in EF in daily life activities do not necessarily have to reside in the brain or specifically in the PFC. Indeed, ratings of EF deficits in daily life activities may be even more sensitive to such detrimental effects of psychiatric disorders or even transient effects of psychologically or emotionally traumatic events than are EF tests.

The existence of deficits at one level of EF are not necessarily contingent on deficits being found at lower levels in the hierarchy of EF, discussed in Barkley (2012b). They can arise at higher levels of EF through various non-neurological influences that can affect the effective utilization of EF at that higher level. Likewise, the existence of EF deficits at a lower level does not automatically ensure their expression at higher levels given that phenotypic expression at that higher level can be dependent on or moderated by the existence of compensatory external structures or environmental factors at that higher level. The long-standing one-level (instrumental–cognitive), one-origin (the brain PFC) perspective of EF deficits is a gross oversimplification and an erroneous one in view of the accumulating evidence not only for the hierarchical organization of EF but also in view of the extended phenotypic effects of EF at a distance. These can be expressed into the expanding and larger spheres of individual daily adaptive functioning, interpersonal social relations, and effective performance in most domains of major life activities over weeks, months, or years of EF performance.

The cognitive level of EF and its underlying linkage to the PFC did not arise in human evolution to take simplistic, short-interval, and socially and emotionally neutered EF tests. It was most likely selected in view of the adaptive problems that arose in human daily life activities most often involving other self-regulating human competitors and cooperators as a means of addressing those adaptive problems (Barkley, 2001, 2012b). Ratings of EF in daily life activities are more likely to detect such extended phenotypic effects than are EF tests or batteries of such tests given their far wider ascertainment window (months vs. minutes), reliance on others who know the child well (parents), greater capacity to capture more environmental settings and domains of major life activities, greater ability to easily incorporate the social and emotional nature of EF, and greater capacity to assess more hierarchically complex and temporally extended EF activities than will ever prove the case for EF tests. As a consequence, more EF deficits in daily life are likely to be found across more neurological and psychiatric disorders or even more psychologically compromising situations on EF ratings than has heretofore been documented using EF tests.

This easily explains the situation that has arisen in the clinical assessment of EF wherein examiners have been more likely to document EF deficits in various neurological and non-neurological disorders using EF ratings than EF tests. Such findings are not cause for frustration with the EF ratings or evidence against the ratings as if they falsely overdocument EF deficits that do not otherwise exist. They are just as easily seen as evidence that indicts the gross undersensitivity of EF cognitive tests to the extended phenotypic expression of EF in important daily life activities over long spans of time in important domains of human adaptive functioning. And such findings for EF ratings also provide evidence that even non-neurological disorders or transient psychological events may affect the expression or effective utilization of EF in daily life activities even if the underlying neurological system that gives rise to EF is itself intact.

To reiterate, EF is a neuropsychological construct that does not depend for its existence and utility as such on some obsessively slavish linkage to a lower biological level of analysis (brain damage) or to some consensus-ordained lab test(s) heralded as the sine qua non of EF. It can be studied for its utility and contribution to understanding human behavior and affairs in its own right independent of the field of neurology. We can do so provided that EF is operationally defined at its own neuropsychological level of analysis and that theoretical models of it at that level are testable, as well as scientifically and clinically useful. EF ratings (and other observational methodologies) have as valuable or more valuable a role to play in such conceptualizations, model building, and testing as do EF tests, as well as in the clinical and scientific evaluation of EF. It should be the evidence available, as well as the level of analysis and extended phenotypic domain of interest to the examiner, that determines the best means by which to assess EF and not some dogmatic adherence to a historically dated obsession with laboratory testing as the gold standard for the evaluation of EF.

Interpreting the BDEFS-CA

The competent professional interpretation of the results of the BDEFS-CA begins with a thorough understanding on the part of the examiner of the nature of EF and its component dimensions. Although Chapter 1 can serve as an introduction to this topic, it is not a substitute for a more thorough grounding in the larger literature on EF. It is therefore essential that the examiner have not only a thorough understanding of the earlier chapters of this manual but also familiarity with the neuropsychological literature on EF, especially as it is manifested in daily life activities (see Barkley, 2012b).

In brief, the BDEFS-CA is intended to measure the capacity of the individual to engage in self-regulation across time for the attainment of future goals, especially in social contexts, and often using social or cultural means to do so. Specifically, the BDEFS-CA evaluates those neuropsychological abilities that serve to support and contribute to this cross-temporal self-regulation toward the future, including Self-Management to Time, Self-Organization/Problem Solving, Self-Restraint (Self-Inhibition), Self-Motivation, and the Self-Regulation of Emotions. Some interpretive information was given earlier in discussing how to score the BDEFS-CA. Further interpretation of the scale is based on the following approaches to understanding the meaning of the scores:

Face Validity

This approach to interpretation is aided by a complete familiarity with the items contained on the scale and the five sections (subscales) to which those items have been assigned. High scores on each scale (typically at or above the 93rd percentile and especially at or above the 98th) may signal a deficiency in this area of EF in daily life activities. One initial means of interpreting each scale in a clinical report is on the basis of the face validity of that subscale. The examiner can actually interpret the meaning of the scale score from the name given to that scale (Self-Management to Time, Self-Organization/Problem Solving, etc.). This interpretation can be enhanced by selecting the individual items from that subscale on which the respondent has scored a 3 or 4 (a symptom) and directly quoting these items in reporting on the meaning of that scale. Given that the scales are moderately to highly intercorrelated, it is most unlikely that an individual will produce deviant scores in just one or two subscales of the BDEFS-CA. Although not impossible, an occurrence in which only a single scale contained a clinically significant score would be cause for further exploration of the reason for such an unusual event. One possibility may be a very discrete, focal brain lesion in a small area of the PFC or cerebellum.

Another would be malingering by the parent or child. A third might be the existence of a highly focal learning disorder such as reading or spelling disorders that might affect just one scale (e.g., Self-Organization/Problem Solving). Also in view of this interrelatedness of the scales, computing interscale differences is not encouraged, as the meaning of disparities across the scales has not been explored in any research to date. This does not mean, however, that relative fluctuations across the scales will not be evident—only that interpretation of the meaning of large disparities between scales has no empirical basis at this time. Just interpreting the meaning of each scale separately is likely to be sufficient to convey the meaning of the BDEFS-CA scores rather than trying to torture the score comparisons to yield up more information than exists about them at the present time.

Normative Comparisons

Further interpretation of each subscale score continues with the comparison of the individual's scores to those of the normative population using the EF Profiles and the resulting percentiles obtained for them in the Appendix. This is then reported as the relative position of the individual in comparison with the general population of children and specifically with the sex and age groups in which they place and the norms used to obtain the percentile score. In short, using the percentile score, the individual is said to place at or above this percentage of individuals in the general population of their age group and sex in their EF in daily life activities.

Risk Analysis (Using the Evidence on Criterion Validity)

As discussed in Chapters 7 and 8, high scores on the BDEFS-CA subscales were associated with a variety of psychiatric disorders, risks for various treatments, and other difficulties in various domains of major life activities. Therefore, the higher the scores observed on the BDEFS-CA, the more likely the child is to be at risk for problems in these same domains of life activities. These risks should be noted in the clinical interpretation of the larger meaning of the BDEFS-CA scores beyond their simply reflecting the five dimensions of EF in daily life for which the subscales are named. Problems with educational, family, peer, and community functioning and various forms of psychological distress or psychiatric disorders (ADHD, BPD, ODD, etc.) were all correlates of higher BDEFS-CA scores that deserve notice by the examiner and probably should be conveyed to the parent where appropriate and applicable. Such information can also be linked to what is already known about the child from the larger evaluation, in which the BDEFS-CA should serve as simply one component when used for a clinical evaluation of a patient. The examiner will have information on the history of the child with regard to these and other major domains of life activity that can serve to place the findings from the BDEFS-CA in this larger context. The BDEFS-CA results can perhaps provide additional hypotheses or even explanations as to the reason that adverse events in these various domains may have been a consequence of or at least associated with deficits in EF. This risk analysis concerning impairments can be further aided by using the BFIS-CA (Barkley, 2012a), for which national norms are available for parent ratings of potential impairment in 15 major domains of children's daily life activities.

Pre- to Postinjury Status

As noted previously, another approach to interpreting the BDEFS-CA exists when the scale has been used to assess possible changes in an individual secondary to a neurological injury or in conjunction with the onset of an acute adverse psychiatric or psychological event. If the BDEFS-CA was given twice to a parent of a child patient with instructions to complete one version for preinjury status and the other postinjury, then these comparisons can be interpreted with appropriate caution for the information they may provide on the impact of the event on EF deficits in daily life activities.

Pre- to Posttreatment Change

As discussed, the BDEFS-CA can also be used to evaluate possible response to intervention by giving the scale to parents before and after an intervention has been implemented with their child. Guidelines were given in this chapter and in Tables 9.1 and 9.2 about how to interpret a change in scores as reflecting reliable change and recovery or normalization. This information can be included in the interpretation of the meaning of the BDEFS-CA scores so obtained.

Conclusion

The BDEFS-CA provides a clinically informative means of evaluating deficits in EF as reported by parents in daily life activities of their children ages 6–17 years. Both a comprehensive 70-item long form and a shorter 20-item version are provided here that can serve to evaluate deficits in EF in the daily life activities of children or adolescents along five interrelated dimensions of EF deficits: Self-Management to Time, Self-Organization/Problem Solving, Self-Restraint, Self-Motivation, and Self-Regulation of Emotion. Further research on and clinical experience with the BDEFS-CA is strongly encouraged. Meanwhile, evidence to date shows the BDEFS-CA to be reasonably reliable, valid, and useful in assessing these dimensions of EF in the daily life activities of children or teenagers. It does so by a means that is efficient and cost-effective. It also yields valuable information on the ways in which these deficits in EF may relate to potential impairments in a variety of domains of major life activities. The adaptive meaningfulness of the BDEFS-CA is documented in its association with impairment in a variety of domains of major life activities in children and adolescents beyond simply documenting the existence of such EF deficits. The scale can be used in clinical practice, research, and educational/organizational settings or in other such venues in which the evaluation of potential deficits in EF in the daily life activities of children or teenagers is of interest. It can also serve as a basis for evaluating change in such deficits, whether as a consequence of treatment or secondary to the occurrence of various neurological and psychiatric disorders or even transient psychological events believed to potentially adversely affect a child's performance in daily life activities. As with the adult version of this scale, I hope that you find these scales useful in your practice.

APPENDIX

BDEFS-CA Forms, Interview, and EF Profiles

BDEFS-CA Long Form

Child's name: ______________________ Date: ______________

Sex: (Circle one) Male Female Age: ______________

Name of person completing this form: ______________________

Relationship to this child: Mother Father Stepmother Stepfather Other (specify): ______________

Instructions

How often does your child experience each of these problems? Please circle the number next to each item that best describes his/her behavior **DURING THE PAST 6 MONTHS**. If your child is currently taking medication for any psychiatric or psychological disorder, please rate his/her behavior based on how he/she acts while **OFF the medication**. Please do not write in the shaded rows that say "Office Use Only."

Section 1 Items	Never or rarely	Some-times	Often	Very often
EF1. Procrastinates or puts off doing things until the last minute	1	2	3	4
EF2. Has a poor sense of time	1	2	3	4
EF3. Wastes or doesn't manage his/her time well	1	2	3	4
EF4. Not prepared on time for schoolwork or assigned tasks given at home	1	2	3	4
EF5. Has trouble planning ahead or preparing for upcoming events	1	2	3	4
EF6. Can't seem to accomplish the goals he/she sets for him/herself	1	2	3	4
EF7. Not able to get things done unless there is an immediate deadline or consequence	1	2	3	4
EF8. Has difficulty judging how much time it will take to do something or get somewhere	1	2	3	4
EF9. Has trouble starting the work he/she is asked to do	1	2	3	4
EF10. Has difficulty sticking with his/her work and getting it done	1	2	3	4
EF11. Not able to prepare in advance for things he/she knows he/she is supposed to do	1	2	3	4
EF12. Has trouble following through on what he/she agrees to do	1	2	3	4
EF13. Has difficulty doing the work he/she is asked to do in the order of its priority or importance; can't "prioritize" well	1	2	3	4
Office Use Only—**Section 1 Total Score** _____				

(cont.)

Section 2 Items	Never or rarely	Some-times	Often	Very often
EF14. When shown something complicated to do, he/she cannot keep it in mind so as to do it correctly	1	2	3	4
EF15. Has trouble considering various ways of doing things	1	2	3	4
EF16. Has difficulty saying what he/she wants to say	1	2	3	4
EF17. Unable to come up with or invent as many solutions to problems as others	1	2	3	4
EF18. At a loss for words when he/she wants to explain something	1	2	3	4
EF19. Has trouble explaining his/her ideas as well or as quickly as others	1	2	3	4
EF20. Not as creative or inventive as others of his/her age	1	2	3	4
EF21. Has trouble learning new or complex activities	1	2	3	4
EF22. Has difficulty explaining things in their proper order or sequence	1	2	3	4
EF23. Can't seem to get to the point of his/her explanations	1	2	3	4
EF24. Has trouble doing things in his/her proper order or sequence	1	2	3	4
EF25. Unable to "think on his/her feet," problem-solve, or respond effectively to unexpected events	1	2	3	4
EF26. Slow at solving problems he/she encounters in his/her daily life	1	2	3	4
EF27. Doesn't seem to process information quickly or accurately	1	2	3	4
Office Use Only—**Section 2 Total Score** _____				
Section 3 Items	Never or rarely	Some-times	Often	Very often
EF28. Has difficulty waiting for things; has to have things or do things he/she wants right away	1	2	3	4
EF29. Makes decisions impulsively	1	2	3	4
EF30. Unable to inhibit his/her reactions to events or to what others say or do to him/her; reacts on impulse	1	2	3	4
EF31. Has difficulty stopping what he/she is doing when it is time to do so	1	2	3	4
EF32. Has difficulty correcting his/her behavior when he/she is given feedback about his/her mistakes	1	2	3	4
EF33. Makes impulsive comments	1	2	3	4
EF34. Likely to do things without considering the consequences for doing them	1	2	3	4
EF35. Acts without thinking things over	1	2	3	4
EF36. Finds it hard to take another person's perspective about a problem or situation	1	2	3	4

(cont.)

EF37. Doesn't stop and talk things over with him/herself before deciding to do something	1	2	3	4
EF38. Has trouble following the rules in a situation	1	2	3	4
EF39. Engages in risky behavior or risk taking	1	2	3	4
EF40. Has trouble with self-discipline (self-control)	1	2	3	4
Office Use Only—**Section 3 Total Score** ______				
Section 4 Items	Never or rarely	Some-times	Often	Very often
EF41. Takes short cuts in his/her chores, schoolwork, or other assignments and does not do all that he/she is supposed to do	1	2	3	4
EF42. Quits working if his/her chores, schoolwork, or other assignments are boring for him/her to do	1	2	3	4
EF43. Does not put much effort into his/her chores, schoolwork, or other assignments	1	2	3	4
EF44. Seems lazy or unmotivated	1	2	3	4
EF45. Has to depend on other people to help get his/her chores, schoolwork, or other assignments done	1	2	3	4
EF46. Things must have an immediate payoff for him/her or he/she is not able to get them done	1	2	3	4
EF47. Has difficulty resisting the urge to do something fun or more interesting when he/she is supposed to be working	1	2	3	4
EF48. Inconsistent in the quality or quantity of his/her work performance	1	2	3	4
EF49. Unable to work without supervision or frequent instruction	1	2	3	4
EF50. Lacks willpower or self-determination	1	2	3	4
EF51. Not able to work toward longer-term or delayed rewards	1	2	3	4
EF52. Not able to resist doing things that produce immediate rewards even if they are not good for him/her in the long run	1	2	3	4
EF53. Gives up too easily if something requires much effort	1	2	3	4
EF54. Not able to get started on his/her chores, school projects, or work without a lot of prodding or encouragement from others	1	2	3	4
Office Use Only—Section 4 Total Score ______				
Section 5 Items	Never or rarely	Some-times	Often	Very often
EF55. Has a low tolerance for frustrating situations	1	2	3	4
EF56. Cannot inhibit his/her emotions	1	2	3	4
EF57. Quick to get angry or become upset	1	2	3	4
EF58. Overreact emotionally	1	2	3	4

(cont.)

EF59. Easily excitable	1	2	3	4
EF60. Not able to inhibit showing strong negative or positive emotions	1	2	3	4
EF61. Has trouble calming him/herself down once he/she is emotionally upset	1	2	3	4
EF62. Not able to be reasonable once he/she is emotional	1	2	3	4
EF63. Cannot seem to distract him/herself away from whatever is upsetting him/her emotionally to help calm down. Can't refocus his/her mind to a more positive framework.	1	2	3	4
EF64. Not able to manage his/her emotions in order to accomplish his/her goals successfully or get along well with others	1	2	3	4
EF65. Remains emotional or upset longer than other children	1	2	3	4
EF66. Finds it difficult to walk away from emotionally upsetting encounters with others or leave situations in which he/she has become very emotional	1	2	3	4
EF67. Not able to rechannel or redirect his/her emotions into more positive ways or outlets when he/she gets upset	1	2	3	4
EF68. Not able to evaluate an emotionally upsetting event more objectively or reasonably	1	2	3	4
EF69. Not able to reevaluate or redefine negative events into a more positive viewpoint when he/she feels strong emotions	1	2	3	4
EF70. Emotionally impulsive or quick to show or express his/her feelings	1	2	3	4
Office Use Only—**Section 5 Total Score** _____				
Office Use Only **Total of Sections 1–5: EF Summary Score** _____ **EF Symptom Count** _____ **[Number of Answers of 3 (Often) or 4 (Very Often)]**				
ADHD-EF Index Score _____ **[Add Items 5, 20, 21, 23, 27, 35, 47, 51, 59, and 68]**				

BDEFS-CA Short Form

Child's name: ______________________________ Date: ______________

Sex: (Circle one) Male Female Age: ______________

Name of person completing this form: ______________________________

Relationship to this child: Mother Father Stepmother Stepfather Other (specify): ______________

Instructions

How often does your child experience each of these problems? Please circle the number next to each item that best describes his/her behavior **DURING THE PAST 6 MONTHS**. If your child is currently taking medication for any psychiatric or psychological disorder, please rate his/her behavior based on how he/she acts while **OFF the medication**. Please do not write in the shaded rows that say "Office Use Only."

Items	Never or rarely	Some-times	Often	Very often
EF1. Procrastinates or puts off doing things until the last minute	1	2	3	4
EF2. Has a poor sense of time	1	2	3	4
EF3. Wastes or doesn't manage his/her time well	1	2	3	4
EF4. Has trouble planning ahead or preparing for upcoming events	1	2	3	4
EF5. Has trouble explaining his/her ideas as well or as quickly as others	1	2	3	4
EF6. Has difficulty explaining things in their proper order or sequence	1	2	3	4
EF7. Can't seem to get to the point of his/her explanations	1	2	3	4
EF8. Doesn't seem to process information quickly or accurately	1	2	3	4
EF9. Makes impulsive comments	1	2	3	4
EF10. Likely to do things without considering the consequences for doing them	1	2	3	4
EF11. Acts without thinking things over	1	2	3	4
EF12. Doesn't stop and talk things over with him/herself before deciding to do something	1	2	3	4
EF13. Takes short cuts in his/her chores, schoolwork, or other assignments and does not do all that he/she is supposed to do	1	2	3	4
EF14. Does not put much effort into his/her chores, schoolwork, or other assignments	1	2	3	4
EF15. Seems lazy or unmotivated	1	2	3	4

(cont.)

EF16. Inconsistent in the quality or quantity of his/her work performance	1	2	3	4
EF17. Has trouble calming him/herself down once he/she is emotionally upset	1	2	3	4
EF18. Not able to be reasonable once he/she is emotional	1	2	3	4
EF19. Cannot seem to distract him/herself away from whatever is upsetting him/her emotionally to help calm down. Can't refocus his/her mind to a more positive framework.	1	2	3	4
EF20. Not able to rechannel or redirect his/her emotions into more positive ways or outlets when he/she gets upset	1	2	3	4
Office Use Only **EF Summary Score** _____ **EF Symptom Count** _____ **[Number of Answers of 3 (Often) or 4 (Very Often)]**				

BDEFS-CA Interview

Child's name: ______________________ Date: ______________

Sex: (Circle one) Male Female Age: ______________

Name of person completing this form: ______________________

Relationship to this child: Mother Father Stepmother Stepfather Other (specify): ______________

Instructions to Interviewer

Say the following to the person to be interviewed: "I would like to ask you a number of questions about your child's behavior during the past 6 months. For each behavior I ask you about, I want to know if it occurs often or more frequently." If your child is currently taking medication for any psychiatric or psychological disorder, please rate his/her behavior based on how he/she acts while **OFF the medication**.

Place a check mark (✓) in the box after each item indicating the answer of the person being interviewed. Each item is simply answered Yes or No.

Interview Questions	No, this does not occur often	Yes, this occurs often or very often
EF1. Procrastinates or puts off doing things until the last minute		
EF2. Has a poor sense of time		
EF3. Wastes or doesn't manage his/her time well		
EF4. Has trouble planning ahead or preparing for upcoming events		
EF5. Has trouble explaining his/her ideas as well or as quickly as others		
EF6. Has difficulty explaining things in their proper order or sequence		
EF7. Can't seem to get to the point of his/her explanations		
EF8. Doesn't seem to process information quickly or accurately		
EF9. Makes impulsive comments		
EF10. Likely to do things without considering the consequences for doing them		
EF11. Acts without thinking things over		
EF12. Doesn't stop and talk things over with him/herself before deciding to do something		
EF13. Takes short cuts in his/her chores, schoolwork, or other assignments and does not do all that he/she is supposed to do		

(cont.)

EF14. Does not put much effort into his/her chores, schoolwork, or other assignments		
EF15. Seems lazy or unmotivated		
EF16. Inconsistent in the quality or quantity of his/her work performance		
EF17. Has trouble calming him/herself down once he/she is emotionally upset		
EF18. Not able to be reasonable once he/she is emotional		
EF19. Cannot seem to distract him/herself away from whatever is upsetting him/her emotionally to help calm down. Can't refocus his/her mind to a more positive framework.		
EF20. Not able to rechannel or redirect his/her emotions into more positive ways or outlets when he/she gets upset		
Office Use Only **Interview Score** _____ **EF Symptom Count** _____		

BDEFS-CA Long Form EF Profile (Ages 6–11, Males Only)

Name: ______________________ Age: ________ Sex: ________ Date: ____________

Raw Scores and Percentiles for Each Subscale

%	Self-Management to Time	Self-Organize	Self-Restraint	Self-Motivate	Self-Regulate Emotion	EF Summary Score	ADHD-EF Index	EF Symptom Count	%
99+	51–52	49–56	50–52	55–56	62–64	248–280	34–40	64–70	99+
98	49–50	43–48	48–49	51–54	59–61	231–247	31–33	60–63	98
97	47–48	40–42	45–47	49–50	56–58	224–230	30	56–59	97
96	45–46	36–39	42–44	46–48	55	210–223	28–29	53–55	96
95	43–44	34–35	40–41	44–45	53–54	202–209	27	50–52	95
94	40–42	33	—	42–43	49–52	196–201	26	44–49	94
93	39	32	39	41	48	188–195	—	42–43	93
92	38	31	37–38	40	47	183–187	25	38–41	92
91	37	—	—	38–39	46	180–182	24	36–37	91
90	36	30	35–36	37	44–45	172–179	23	33–35	90
89	35	29	34	36	42–43	171	—	31–32	89
88	—	28	33	35	41	165–170	22	29–30	88
87	34	—	32	34	40	162–164	—	28	87
86	33	—	31	—	38–39	158–161	21	26–27	86
85	32	27	30	33	—	153–157	—	25	85
84	31	26	29	32	37	150–152	20	23–24	84
83	—	—	—	—	—	148–149	—	22	83
82	—	25	—	31	36	146–147	—	20–21	82
81	30	—	28	30	35	144–145	—	19	81
80	—	—	—	—	34	143	—	17–18	80
79	29	24	—	—	33	140–142	—	16	79
78	—	23	27	29	—	—	19	15	78
77	—	—	—	—	—	139	—	—	77
76	28	22	—	28	32	138	—	14	76
75	—	—	26	—	—	137	—	13	75
74	27	—	—	—	—	135–136	18	12	74
73	—	—	—	—	—	133–134	—	—	73
72	—	21	—	—	—	132	—	11	72
71	—	—	—	—	31	130–131	—	—	71
70	26	—	—	—	—	128–129	17	10	70
60–69	24–25	19–20	24–25	25–27	26–30	119–127	16	5–9	60–69
50–59	23	17–18	22–23	22–24	24–25	111–118	15	2–4	50–59
40–49	21–22	16	18–21	19–21	21–23	98–110	13–14	1	40–49
30–39	18–20	15	16–17	17–18	19–20	91–97	—	0	30–39
20–29	16–17	14	15	15–16	17–18	82–90	11–12	—	20–29
10–19	14–15	—	13–14	14	16	73–81	10	—	10–19
1–9	13	—	—	—	—	70–72	—	—	1–9
Raw Score									Raw Score

Sample size = 451

Note. Self-Organize, Self-Organizational/Problem Solving; Self-Motivate, Self-Motivation; Self-Regulate Emotion, Self-Regulation of Emotion.

BDEFS-CA Long Form EF Profile (Ages 12–17, Males Only)

Name: ______________________ Age: ________ Sex: ________ Date: __________

Raw Scores and Percentiles for Each Subscale

%	Self-Management to Time	Self-Organize	Self-Restraint	Self-Motivate	Self-Regulate Emotions	EF Summary Score	ADHD-EF Index	EF Symptom Count	%
99+	52	52–56	51–52	55–56	64	258–280	36–40	67–70	99+
98	50–51	44–51	49–50	53–54	59–63	239–257	34–35	63–66	98
97	49	42–43	46–48	52	56–58	227–238	32–33	60–62	97
96	47–48	40–41	44–45	50–51	51–55	217–226	30–31	56–59	96
95	44–46	39	42–43	49	49–50	210–216	—	53–55	95
94	43	37–38	40–41	47–48	45–48	201–209	29	48–52	94
93	42	36	38–39	45–46	43–44	199–200	27–28	45–47	93
92	40–41	35	36–37	44	41–42	189–198	26	43–44	92
91	—	33–34	—	43	40	184–188	25	41–42	91
90	39	32	34–35	42	39	181–183	24	37–40	90
89	—	31	—	41	38	179–180	—	34–36	89
88	38	30	32–33	40	37	173–178	23	31–33	88
87	37	29	—	—	36	166–172	22	30	87
86	36	28	31	38–39	—	159–165	—	27–29	86
85	35	—	30	36–37	34–35	156–158	21	25–26	85
84	—	—	29	35	—	152–155	—	24	84
83	—	—	—	34	33	150–151	—	22–23	83
82	34	—	28	—	—	149	20	21	82
81	—	27	—	33	32	148	—	20	81
80	33	—	27	—	—	146–147	—	18–19	80
79	—	—	—	32	—	144–145	—	—	79
78	—	26	26	—	—	142–143	—	17	78
77	—	25	—	—	—	141	—	16	77
76	32	24	—	31	31	140	19	—	76
75	31	23	—	—	—	—	—	14–15	75
74	30	—	—	30	30	138–139	—	13	74
73	—	—	25	29	29	—	—	—	73
72	—	—	—	—	—	134–137	18	12	72
71	—	22	—	—	—	133	—	—	71
70	29	21	24	—	28	132	—	11	70
60–69	26–28	19–20	21–23	25–28	24–27	116–131	16–17	6–10	60–69
50–59	24–25	17–18	19–20	22–24	21–23	108–115	14–15	3–5	50–59
40–49	22–23	16	17–18	19–21	18–20	97–107	13	1–2	40–49
30–39	19–21	15	16	17–18	17	87–96	12	0	30–39
20–29	16–18	14	14–15	15–16	16	80–86	11	—	20–29
10–19	14–15	—	13	14	—	74–79	10	—	10–19
1–9	13	—	—	—	—	70–73	—	—	1–9
Raw Score									Raw Score

Sample size = 450

Note. Self-Organize, Self-Organizational/Problem Solving; Self-Motivate, Self-Motivation; Self-Regulate Emotion, Self-Regulation of Emotion.

BDEFS-CA Long Form EF Profile (Ages 6–11, Females Only)

Name: ______________________ Age: ________ Sex: ________ Date: ____________

Raw Scores and Percentiles for Each Subscale

%	Self-Management to Time	Self-Organize	Self-Restraint	Self-Motivate	Self-Regulate Emotions	EF Summary Score	ADHD-EF Index	EF Symptom Count	%
99+	48–52	48–56	49–52	52–56	62–64	234–280	34–40	64–70	99+
98	44–47	41–47	45–48	48–51	59–61	213–233	30–33	53–63	98
97	43	36–40	41–44	46–47	53–58	203–212	29	48–52	97
96	39–42	34–35	38–40	44–45	50–52	193–202	26–28	42–47	96
95	—	33	36–37	43	48–49	183–192	—	37–41	95
94	37–38	31–32	34–35	39–42	45–47	175–182	24–25	34–36	94
93	36	30	33	36–38	44	172–174	23	31–33	93
92	—	29	32	35	43	165–171	22	30	92
91	35	28	31	34	—	161–164	—	28–29	91
90	33–34	—	—	33	42	160	—	26–27	90
89	—	—	—	32	41	157–159	21	24–25	89
88	32	27	29–30	31	40	153–156	—	22–23	88
87	31	26	—	—	39	150–152	20	20–21	87
86	—	—	28	30	38	147–149	—	19	86
85	30	25	27	29	36–37	145–146	—	17–18	85
84	29	24	—	—	—	142–144	19	—	84
83	—	—	26	28	35	140–141	—	16	83
82	28	—	—	—	34	138–139	—	14–15	82
81	—	23	—	—	33	136–137	—	13	81
80	27	22	25	27	—	134–135	18	12	80
79	—	—	—	—	—	—	—	11	79
78	—	—	—	26	32	132–133	—	10	78
77	26	21	—	—	—	130–131	—	9	77
76	—	—	24	25	31	127–129	—	—	76
75	—	—	—	—	—	125–126	17	8	75
74	—	—	—	—	30	123–124	—	7	74
73	25	—	—	—	—	122	—	—	73
72	—	20	23	24	29	121	—	6	72
71	—	—	—	—	—	119–120	—	—	71
70	—	—	22	—	28	—	16	5	70
60–69	23–24	18–19	20–21	21–23	24–27	107–118	15	2–4	60–69
50–59	21–22	16–17	18–19	19–20	21–23	98–106	13–14	1	50–59
40–49	19–20	15	16–17	17–18	19–20	89–97	12	0	40–49
30–39	17–18	14	15	15–16	17–18	84–88	11	—	30–39
20–29	15–16	—	13–14	14	16	78–83	—	—	20–29
10–19	13–14	—	—	—	—	72–77	10	—	10–19
1–9	—	—	—	—	—	70–71	—	—	1–9
Raw Score									Raw Score

Sample size = 451

Note. Self-Organize, Self-Organizational/Problem Solving; Self-Motivate, Self-Motivation; Self-Regulate Emotion, Self-Regulation of Emotion.

BDEFS-CA Long Form EF Profile (Ages 12–17, Females Only)

Name: ____________________ Age: ________ Sex: ________ Date: ________

Raw Scores and Percentiles for Each Subscale

%	Self-Management to Time	Self-Organize	Self-Restraint	Self-Motivate	Self-Regulate Emotions	EF Summary Score	ADHD-EF Index	EF Symptom Count	%
99+	51–52	46–52	49–52	52–56	62–64	233–264	31–40	58–70	99+
98	47–50	39–45	44–48	50–51	59–61	208–232	29–30	49–57	98
97	44–46	36–38	43	45–49	53–58	200–207	27–28	47–48	97
96	41–43	34–35	41–42	44	47–52	192–199	26	40–46	96
95	39–40	33	37–40	40–43	46	180–191	25	36–39	95
94	38	32	35–36	38–39	43–45	176–179	—	35	94
93	37	31	—	37	—	173–175	24	33–34	93
92	36	30	34	36	41–42	171–172	23	32	92
91	35	29	32–33	35	39–40	166–170	22	30–31	91
90	—	—	31	—	38	163–165	—	28–29	90
89	34	28	30	34	37	159–162	—	26–27	89
88	—	—	29	33	36	156–158	21	24–25	88
87	33	—	28	32	35	154–155	—	22–23	87
86	32	27	—	31	—	152–153	20	—	86
85	—	—	27	—	34	148–151	—	20–21	85
84	31	26	—	30	33	145–147	—	19	84
83	30	25	26	—	—	141–144	—	18	83
82	—	—	—	29	32	140	19	17	82
81	—	24	25	—	—	139	—	16	81
80	—	23	—	28	31	138	—	14–15	80
79	29	—	—	—	—	137	18	13	79
78	28	—	—	—	—	134–136	—	12	78
77	—	22	24	27	—	133	—	11	77
76	—	—	—	—	—	132	17	10	76
75	27	—	—	—	30	130–131	—	8–9	75
74	—	21	—	—	—	128–129	—	7	74
73	—	—	23	26	29	127	—	6	73
72	26	—	—	—	—	124–126	—	—	72
71	—	20	—	—	28	120–123	—	—	71
70	—	—	22	—	—	119	—	5	70
60–69	24–25	18–19	20–21	22–25	24–27	108–118	15–16	3–4	60–69
50–59	22–23	16–17	18–19	19–21	21–23	99–107	13–14	1–2	50–59
40–49	19–21	15	16–17	17–18	19–20	91–98	12	0	40–49
30–39	16–18	14	15	15–16	17–18	82–90	11	—	30–39
20–29	15	—	13–14	14	16	76–81	10	—	20–29
10–19	13–14	—	—	—	—	72–75	—	—	10–19
1–9	—	—	—	—	—	70–71	—	—	1–9
Raw Score									Raw Score

Sample size = 448

Note. Self-Organize, Self-Organizational/Problem Solving; Self-Motivate, Self-Motivation; Self-Regulate Emotion, Self-Regulation of Emotion.

BDEFS-CA Short Form EF Profile (All Ages and Both Sexes)

Name: ______________________ Age: ________ Sex: ________ Date: __________

Raw Scores and Percentiles for Each Sex and Age Group

	Males				Females				
	Ages 6–11		Ages 12–17		Ages 6–11		Ages 12–17		
%	EF Summary	EF Symptom Count	EF Summary	EF Symptom Count	EF Summary	EF Symptom Count	EF Summary	EF Symptom Count	%
99+	71–80	19–20	75–80	20	69–80	18–20	69–80	17–20	99+
98	67–70	18	71—74	19	65–68	16–17	62–68	14–16	98
97	64–66	16–17	68–70	18	61–64	15	59–61	13	97
96	60–63	15	64–67	17	57–60	13–14	55–58	—	96
95	58–59	14	62–63	16	54–56	12	54	12	95
94	56–57	13	59–61	15	50–53	10–11	53	11	94
93	54–55	12	57–58	14	49	9	51–52	10	93
92	52–53	11	56	12–13	48	8	50	—	92
91	50–51	10	54–55	—	46–47	—	49	9	91
90	49	—	53	11	—	7	48	8	90
89	48	9	52	10	44–45	—	47	—	89
88	46–47	8	51	—	43	6	46	—	88
87	—	—	49–50	9	—	—	45	7	87
86	45	7	48	—	42	—	—	—	86
85	44	—	47	—	—	5	43–44	—	85
84	43	—	—	8	41	—	—	—	84
83	42	6	46	—	—	—	42	6	83
82	—	—	45	7	40	4	—	—	82
81	—	—	44	—	—	—	41	5	81
80	41	5	—	—	39	—	—	—	80
79	40	—	—	6	—	3	40	—	79
78	—	—	43	—	38	—	—	—	78
77	—	—	42	—	37	—	—	4	77
76	—	4	41	—	—	—	—	—	76
75	39	—	—	5	36	—	39	—	75
74	—	—	40	—	—	—	38	3	74
73	—	—	—	—	35	—	—	—	73
72	38	3	—	—	—	2	—	—	72
71	—	—	39	4	—	—	37	—	71
70	—	—	—	—	34	—	—	2	70
60–69	34–37	2	35–38	2-3	31–33	1	33–36	1	60–69
50–59	32–33	1	32–34	1	29–30	0	29–32	0	50–59
40–49	29–31	0	29–31	0	26–28	—	27–28	—	40–49
30–39	27–28	—	26–28	—	25	—	25–26	—	30–39
20–29	24–26	—	24–25	—	23–24	—	23–24	—	20–29
10–19	21–23	—	22–23	—	20–22	—	21–22	—	10–19
0–9	20	—	20–21	—	—	—	20	—	0–9
Raw Score									Raw Score

References

Achenbach, T. M. (2001). *Manual for the Child Behavior Checklist/4–18 and 1991 Profile.* Burlington, VT: Author.

Airaksinen, E., Larsson, M., & Forsell, Y. (2005). Neuropsychological functions in anxiety disorders in population-based samples: Evidence of episodic memory dysfunction. *Journal of Psychiatric Research, 39,* 207–214.

Alderman, N., Burgess, P. W., Knight, C., & Henman, C. (2003). Ecological validity of a simplified version of the Multiple Errands Shopping Test. *Journal of the International Neuropsychological Society, 9,* 31–44.

American Psychiatric Association. (2000). *Diagnostic and statistical manual of mental disorders* (4th ed., tex rev.). Washington, DC: Author.

American Psychological Association. (1999). *The Standards for Education and Psychological Testing.* Washington, DC: Author.

Anderson, P. (2002). Assessment and development of executive function (EF) during childhood. *Child Neuropsychology, 8,* 71–82.

Anderson, V. A., Anderson, P., Northam, E., Jacobs, R., & Mikiewicz, O. (2002). Relationships between cognitive and behavioral measures of executive function in children with brain disease. *Child Neuropsychology, 8,* 231–240.

Ardila, A., & Surloff, C. (2006). Dysexecutive agraphia: A major executive dysfunction sign. *International Journal of Neuroscience, 116,* 653–663.

Baddeley, A. (1986). *Working memory.* Oxford, UK: Clarendon Press.

Baddeley, A. D., & Hitch, G. J. (1994). Developments in the concept of working memory. *Neuropsychology, 8,* 485–493.

Banaschewski, T., Neale, B. M., Rothenberger, A., & Roessner, V. (2007). Comorbidity of tic disorders and ADHD: Conceptual and methodological considerations. *European Child and Adolescent Psychiatry, 16*(Suppl. 1), 5–14.

Barkley, R. A. (1988). Child behavior rating scales and checklists. In M. Rutter, H. A. Tuma, & I. S. Lann (Eds.), *Assessment and diagnosis in child psychopathology* (pp. 113–155). New York: Guilford Press.

Barkley, R. A. (1991). The ecological validity of laboratory and analogue assessments of ADHD symptoms. *Journal of Abnormal Child Psychology, 19,* 149–178.

Barkley, R. A. (1994). Impaired delayed responding: A unified theory of attention deficit hyperactivity disorder. In D. K. Routh (Ed.), *Disruptive behavior disorders in childhood: Essays honoring Herbert C. Quay* (pp. 11–57). New York: Plenum.

Barkley, R. A. (1997a). *ADHD and the nature of self-control.* New York: Guilford Press.

Barkley, R. A. (1997b). *Defiant children: A clinician's manual for parent training.* New York: Guilford Press.

Barkley, R. A. (1997c). Inhibition, sustained attention, and executive functions: Constructing a unifying theory of ADHD. *Psychological Bulletin, 121,* 65–94.

Barkley, R. A. (2001). Executive functions and self-regulation: An evolutionary neuropsychological perspective. *Neuropsychology Review, 11,* 1–29.

Barkley, R. A. (2006). *Attention-deficit hyperactivity disorder: A handbook for diagnosis and treatment* (3rd ed.) New York: Guilford Press.

Barkley, R. A. (2010). Deficient emotional self-regulation is a core component of ADHD. *Journal of ADHD and Related Disorders, 1,* 5–37.

Barkley, R. A. (2011a). *Barkley Deficits in Executive Functioning Scale* (BDEFS). New York: Guilford Press.

Barkley, R. A. (2011b). *Barkley Functional Impairment Scale (BFIS).* New York: Guilford Press.

Barkley, R. A. (2012a). *Barkley Functional Impairment Scale—Children and Adolescents (BFIS-CA).* New York: Guilford Press.

Barkley, R. A. (2012b). *Executive functions: What they are, how they work, and why they evolved.* New York: Guilford Press.

Barkley, R. A. (in press). Distinguishing sluggish cognitive tempo from attention deficit hyperactivity disorder symptoms in adults. *Journal of Abnormal Psychology.*

Barkley, R. A., & Fischer, M. (2011). Predicting impairment in occupational functioning in hyperactive children as adults: Self-reported executive function (EF) deficits vs. EF tests. *Developmental Neuropsychology, 36,* 137–161.

Barkley, R. A., Knouse, L. E., & Murphy, K. R. (2011). Correspondence and disparity in the self and other ratings of current and childhood symptoms and impairments in adults with ADHD. *Psychological Assessment, 23,* 437–446.

Barkley, R. A., & Murphy, K. R. (2006). *Attention-deficit hyperactivity disorder: A clinical workbook* (3rd ed.). New York: Guilford Press.

Barkley, R. A., & Murphy, K. R. (2010). Impairment in major life activities and adult ADHD: The predictive utility of executive function (EF) ratings vs. EF tests. *Archives of Clinical Neuropsychology, 25,* 157–173.

Barkley, R. A., & Murphy, K. R. (2011). The nature of executive function (EF) deficits in daily life activities in adults with ADHD and their relationship to EF tests. *Journal of Psychopathology and Behavioral Assessment, 33,* 137–158.

Barkley, R. A., Murphy, K. R., DuPaul, G. I., & Bush, T. (2002). Driving in young adults with attention deficit hyperactivity disorder: Knowledge, performance, adverse outcomes, and the role of executive functioning. *Journal of the International Neuropsychological Society, 8,* 655–672.

Barkley, R. A., Murphy, K. R., & Fischer, M. (2008). *ADHD in adults: What the science says.* New York: Guilford Press.

Barnett, R., Maruff, P., & Vance, A. (2009). Neurocognitive function in attention-deficit-hyperactivity disorder with and without comorbid disruptive behavior disorders. *Australian and New Zealand Journal of Psychiatry, 43,* 722–730.

Bekhterev, V. M. (1905–1907). *Fundamentals of brain function.* St. Petersburg, Russia: Brokhauzi Efron.

Bell, M. A., Wolfe, C. D., & Adkins, D. R. (2007). Frontal lobe development during infancy and childhood. In D. Coch, K. W.. Fischer, & G. Dawson (Eds.), *Human behavior, learning, and the developing brain: Typical development* (pp. 247–276). New York: Guilford Press.

Best, J. R., Miller, P. H., & Jones, L. J. (2009). Executive functions after age 5: Changes and correlates. *Developmental Review, 29,* 180–200.

Bianchi, L. (1895). The functions of the frontal lobes. *Brain, 18,* 497–522.

Bianchi, L. (1922). *The mechanism of the brain and the function of the frontal lobes.* Edinburgh, UK: Livingstone.

Biederman, J., Petty, C. R., Fried, R., Black, S., Faneuil, A., Doyle, A. E., et al. (2008). Discordance between psychometric testing and questionnaire-based definitions of executive function deficits in individuals with ADHD. *Journal of Attention Disorders, 12,* 92–102.

Biederman, J., Petty, C. R., Fried, R., Doyle, A. E., Mick, E., Aleardi, M., et al. (2008). Utility of an abbreviated questionnaire to identify individuals with ADHD at risk for functional impairments. *Journal of Psychiatric Research, 42*(4), 304–310.

Black, L., Schefft, B. K., Howe, S. R., Szaflarski, J. P., Yeh, H., & Privitera, M. D. (2010). The effect of seizures on working memory and executive functioning performance. *Epilepsy and Behavior, 17,* 412–419.

Bogod, N. M., Mateer, C. A., & MacDonald, S. W. S. (2003). Self-awareness after traumatic brain injury: A comparison of measures and their relationship to executive functions. *Journal of the International Neuropsychological Society, 9,* 450–458.

Boonstra, A. M., Oosterlaan, J., Sergeant, J. A., & Buitelaar, J. K. (2005). Executive functioning in adult ADHD: A meta-analytic review. *Psychological Medicine, 35,* 1097–1108.

Borkowski, J. G., & Burke, J. E. (1996). Theories, models, and measurements of executive functioning: An information processing perspective. In G. R. Lyon & N. A. Krasnegor (Eds.), *Attention, memory, and executive functioning* (pp. 235–262). Baltimore: Brookes.

Boyle, C. A., Decoufle, P., & Yeargin-Allsop, M. (1994). Prevalence and health impact of developmental disabilities in U.S. children. *Pediatrics, 93,* 399–403.

Brandenburg, N. A., Friedman, R. M., & Silver, S. E. (1990). The epidemiology of childhood psychiatric disorders: Prevalence findings from recent studies. *Journal of the American Academy of Child and Adolescent Psychiatry, 29,* 76–83.

Bronowski, J. (1977). Human and animal languages. In *A sense of the future* (pp. 104–131). Cambridge, MA: MIT Press.

Bryant, F. B. (2000). Assessing the validity of measurement. In. L. G. Grim & P. R. Yarnold (Eds.), *Reading and understanding more multivariate statistics* (pp. 99–146). Washington, DC: American Psychological Association.

Buckholtz, J. W., Treadway, M. T., Cowan, R. L., Woodward, N. D., Li, R., Ansari, M. S., et al. (2010). Dopaminergic network differences in human impulsivity. *Science, 319,* 532.

Burgess, P. W., Alderman, N., Evans, J., Emslie, H., & Wilson, B. A. (1998). The ecological validity of tests of executive function. *Journal of the International Neuropsychological Society, 4,* 547–558.

Bush, G., Valera, E. M., & Seidman, L. J. (2005). Functional neuroimaging of attention-deficit/hyperactivity disorder: A review and suggested future directions. *Biological Psychiatry, 57,* 1273–1296.

Butterfield, E. C., & Albertson, L. R. (1995). On making cognitive theory more general and developmentally pertinent. In F. Weinert & W. Schneider (Eds.), *Research on memory development* (pp. 73–99). Hillsdale, NJ: Erlbaum.

Butterfield, E. C., & Belmont, J. M. (1977). Assessing and improving the executive cognitive functions of mentally retarded persons. In I. Bialer & M. Steinlich (Eds.), *The psychology of mental retardation* (pp. 277–307). New York: Psychological Dimensions.

Cairns, R. B., & Green, J. A. (1979). How to assess personality and social patterns: Observations or ratings? In. R. B. Cairns (Ed.), *The analysis of social interactions* (pp. 209–226). Hillsdale, NJ: Erlbaum.

Capano, L., Minden, D., Chen, S. X., Schachar, R. J., & Ickowicz, A. (2008). Mathematical learning disorder in school-age children with attention-deficit hyperactivity disorder. *Canadian Journal of Psychiatry, 53,* 392–399.

Carlson, G. A., & Meyer, S. E. (2009). ADHD with mood disorders. In T. E. Brown (Ed.), *ADHD comorbidities: Handbook for ADHD complications in children and adults* (pp. 97–130). Washington, DC: American Psychiatric Publishing.

Cartwright-Hatton, S., McNicol, K., & Doubleday, K. (2006). Anxiety in a neglected population: Prevalence of anxiety disorders in pre-adolescent children. *Clinical Psychology Review, 26,* 817–833.

Castellanos, X., Sonuga-Barke, E., Milham, M., & Tannock, R. (2006). Characterizing cognition in ADHD: Beyond executive dysfunction. *Trends in Cognitive Sciences, 10,* 117–123.

Chaytor, N., Schmitter-Edgecombe, M., & Burr, R. (2006). Improving the ecological validity of executive functioning assessment. *Archives of Clinical Neuropsychology, 21,* 217–227.

Ciairano, S., Visu-Petra, L., & Settanni, M. (2007). Executive inhibitory control and cooperative behavior during early school years: A follow-up study. *Journal of Abnormal Child Psychology, 35,* 335–345.

Clements, G. L., Lee, R. H., & Barclay, A. M. (1988). Tic disorders of childhood. *American Family Physician, 38,* 163–170.

Cohen, J. (1992). A power primer. *Psychological Bulletin, 112,* 155–159.

Cook, T. D., & Campbell, D. T. (1979). *Quasi-experimentation: Design and analysis issues for field settings.* Chicago: Rand McNally.

Corbett, B. A., Constantine, L. J., Hendren, R., Rocke, D., & Ozonoff, S. (2009). Examining executive functioning in children with autism spectrum disorder, attention deficit hyperactivity disorder and typical development. *Psychiatry Research, 166,* 210–222.

Costello, E. J., Angold, A., Burns, B. J., Stangl, D. K., Tweed, D. L., Erkanli, A., et al. (1996). The Great Smoky Mountains Study of Youth: Goals, design, methods, and the prevalence of DSM-III-R disorders. *Archives of General Psychiatry, 53,* 1129–1136.

Costello, E. J., Egger, H., & Angold, A. (2005). 10-year research update review: The epidemiology of child and adolescent psychiatric disorders: I. Methods and public health burden. *Journal of the American Academy of Child and Adolescent Psychiatry, 44,* 972–986.

Costello, E. J., Mustillo, S., Erkanli, A., Keeler, G., & Angold, A. (2003). Prevalence and development of psychiatric disorders in childhood and adolescence. *Archives of General Psychiatry, 60,* 837–844.

Culhane-Shelburne, K., Chapieski, L., Hiscock, M., & Glaze, D. (2002). Executive functions in children with frontal and temporal lobe epilepsy. *Journal of the International Neuropsychological Society, 8,* 623–632.

Dawkins, R. (1982). *The extended phenotype.* New York: Oxford University Press.

Del'Homme, M., Kim, T. S., Loo, S. K., Yang, M. H., & Smalley, S. L. (2007). Familial association and frequency of learning disabilities in ADHD sibling pair families. *Journal of Abnormal Child Psychology, 35,* 35–55.

Denckla, M. B. (1996). A theory and model of executive function: a neuropsychological perspective. In G. R. Lyon & N. A. Krasnegor (Eds.), *Attention, memory, and executive function* (pp. 263–278). Baltimore: Brookes.

Dimond, S. J. (1980). *Neuropsychology: A textbook of systems and psychological functions of the human brain.* London: Butterworths.

Dodrill, C. B. (1997). Myths of neuropsychology. *Clinical Neuropsychologist, 11,* 1–17.

Emerson, C. S., Mollet, G. A., & Harrison, D. W. (2005). Anxious-depression in boys: An evaluation of executive functioning. *Archives of Clinical Neuropsychology, 20,* 539–546.

Eslinger, P. J. (1996). Conceptualizing, describing, and measuring components of executive function: A summary. In G. R. Lyon & N. A. Krasnegor (Eds.), *Attention, memory, and executive function* (pp. 367–395). Baltimore: Brookes.

Essau, C. A., Conradt, J., & Petermann, F. (2000). Frequency, comorbidity, and psychosocial impairment of anxiety disorders in German adolescents. *Journal of Anxiety Disorders, 14,* 263–279.

Fedele, D. A., Hartung, C. M., Canu, W. H., & Wilkowski, B. M. (2010). Potential symptoms of ADHD for emerging adults. *Journal of Psychopathology and Behavioral Assessment, 32,* 385–396.

Fleming, J. E., Offord, D. R., & Boyle, M. H. (1989). Prevalence of childhood and adolescent depression in the community: The Ontario Child Health Study. *British Journal of Psychiatry, 155,* 647–654.

Frazier, T. W., Demareem, H. A., & Youngstrom, E. A. (2004). Meta-analysis of intellectual and neuropsychological test performance in attention-deficit/hyperactivity disorder. *Neuropsychology, 18,* 543–555.

Fuster, J. M. (1989). *The prefrontal cortex* (2nd ed.). New York: Raven.

Fuster, J. M. (1997). *The prefrontal cortex* (3rd ed.). Philadelphia: Lippincott-Raven.

Geary, D. C., Hoard, M. K., Byrd-Craven, J., Nugent, L., & Numtee, C. (2007). Cognitive mechanisms underlying achievement deficits in children with mathematical learning disability. *Child Development, 78,* 1343–1359.

Germanò, E., Gagliano, A., & Curatolo, P. (2010). Comorbidity of ADHD and dyslexia. *Developmental Neuropsychology, 35,* 475–493.

Gilotty, L., Kenworthy, L., Sirian, L., Black, D. O., & Wagner, A. E. (2002). Adaptive skills and executive function in autism spectrum disorders. *Child Neuropsychology, 8,* 241–248.

Gioia, G. A., Isquith, P. K., Guy, S. C., & Kenworthy, L. (2000). *BRIEF: Behavior Rating Inventory of Executive Function—Professional manual.* Odessa, FL: Psychological Assessment Resources.

Gioia, G. A., Isquith, P. K., Kenworthy, L., & Barton, R. M. (2002). Profiles of everyday executive function in acquired and developmental disorders. *Child Neuropsychology, 8,* 121–137.

Gottman, J., & Katz, L. (1989). Effects of marital discord on young children's peer interaction and health. *Developmental Psychology, 25,* 373–381.

Goulden, L. G., & Silver, C. H. (2009). Concordance of the Children's Executive Functions Scale with established tests and parent rating scales. *Journal of Psychoeducational Assessment, 27,* 439–451.

Griffith, E. M., Pennington, B. F., Wehner, E. A., & Rogers, S. J. (2003). Executive functions in young children with autism. *Child Development, 70,* 817–832.

Groot, C. M. de, Yeates, K. O., Baker, G. B., & Bornstein, R. A. (1997). Impaired neuropsychological functioning in Tourette's syndrome subjects with co-occurring obsessive–compulsive and attention-deficit symptoms. *Journal of Neuropsychiatry and Clinical Neuroscience, 9,* 267–272.

Gropper, R. J., & Tannock, R. (2009). A pilot study of working memory and academic achievement in college students with ADHD. *Journal of Attention Disorders, 12,* 574–581.

Gross, J. J. (1998). The emerging field of emotion regulation: An integrative review. *Review of General Psychology, 2,* 271–299.

Gross, J. J., & John, O. P. (2003). Individual differences in two emotion regulation processes: Implications for affect, relationships, and well-being. *Journal of Personality and Social Psychology, 85,* 348–362.

Gross, J. J., & Thompson, R. A. (2007). Emotion regulation: Conceptual foundations. In J. J. Gross (Ed.), *Handbook of emotion regulation* (pp. 3–24). New York: Guilford Press.

Gruber, O., & Goschke, T. (2003). Executive control emerging from dynamic interactions between brain systems mediating language, working memory, and attentional processes. *Acta Psychologica, 115,* 105–121.

Guerts, H. G., Verte, S., Oosterlaan, J., Roeyers, H., & Sergeant, J. (2004). How specific are executive functioning deficits in attention deficit disorder and autism? *Journal of Child Psychology and Psychiatry, 45,* 836–854.

Gunther, T., Holtkamp, K., Jolles, J., Herpertz-Dahlmann, B., & Konrad, K. (2004). Verbal memory and aspects of attentional control in children and adolescents with anxiety disorders or depressive disorders. *Journal of Affective Disorders, 82,* 265–269.

Guttmann-Steinmetz, S., Gadow, K. D., De Vincent, C. J., & Crowell, J. (2010). Anxiety symptoms in boys with autism spectrum disorder, attention-deficit hyperactivity disorder, or chronic tic disorder and community controls. *Journal of Autism and Developmental Disorders, 40,* 1006–1016.

Haenlein, M., & Caul, W. F. (1987). Attention deficit disorder with hyperactivity: A specific hypothesis of reward dysfunction. *Journal of the American Academy of Child and Adolescent Psychiatry, 26,* 356–362.

Hammerness, P., Geller, D., Petty, C., Lamb, A., Bristol, E., & Biederman, J. (2010). Does ADHD moderate the manifestation of anxiety disorders in children? *European Child and Adolescent Psychiatry, 19,* 107–112.

Harlow, J. M. (1848). Passage of an iron rod through the head. *Boston Medical and Surgical Journal, 39,* 389–393.

Harlow, J. M. (1868). Recovery from the passage of an iron rod through the head. *Publications of the Massachusetts Medical Society, 2,* 237–346.

Harris, E. L., Schuerholz, L. J., Singer, H. S., Reader, M. J., Brown, J. E., Cox, C., et al. (1995). Executive function in children with Tourette syndrome and/or attention deficit hyperactivity disorder. *Journal of the International Neuropsychological Society, 1,* 511–516.

Hayes, S. C. (1989). *Rule-governed behavior: Cognition, contingencies, and instructional control.* New York: Plenum Press.

Hayes, S. C., Gifford, E. V., & Ruckstuhl, L. E., Jr. (1996). Relational frame theory and executive function: A behavioral approach. In G. R. Lyon & N. A. Krasnegor (Eds.), *Attention, memory, and executive function* (pp. 279–305). Baltimore: Brookes.

Hervey, A. S., Epstein, J. N., & Curry, J. F. (2004). Neuropsychology of adults with attention-deficit/hyperactivity disorder: A meta-analytic review. *Neuropsychology, 18,* 495–503.

Hinshaw, S. P. (2002). Is ADHD an impairing condition in childhood and adolescence? In P. S. Jensen (Ed.), *Attention deficit hyperactivity disorder: State of the science—best practices.* (pp. 5-1–5-21). Kingston, NJ: Civic Research Institute.

Hughes, C., Ensor, R., Wilson, A., & Graham, A. (2010). Tracking executive function across the transition to school: A latent variable approach. *Developmental Neuropsychology, 35,* 20–36.

Huizinga, M., Dolan, C. V., & van der Molen, M. W. (2006). Age-related change in executive function: Developmental trends and a latent variable analysis. *Neuropsychologia, 44,* 2017–2036.

Hummer, T. A., Kronenberger, W. G., Wang, Y., Dunn, D. W., Mosier, K. M., Kalnin, A. J., et al. (2011). Executive functioning characteristics associated with ADHD comorbidity in adolescents with disruptive behavior disorders. *Journal of Abnormal Child Psychology, 39*(1), 11–19.

Hutchinson, A. D., Mathias, J. L., & Banich, M. T. (2008). Corpus callosum morphology in children and adolescents with attention deficit hyperactivity disorder: A meta-analytic review. *Neuropsychology, 22,* 341–349.

Jacobson, N. S., Roberts, L. J., Berns, S. B., & McGlinchey, J. B. (1999). Methods for defining and determining the clinical significance of treatment effects: Description, application, and alternatives. *Journal of Consulting and Clinical Psychology, 67,* 300–307.

Jacobson, N. S., & Truax, P. (1991). Clinical significance: A statistical approach to defining meaningful change in psychotherapy research. *Journal of Consulting and Clinical Psychology, 59,* 12–19.

Jastak, J., & Wilkinson, G. (1993). *The Wide Range Achivement Test—3*. Wilmington, DE: Jastak.

Jong, C. G. W. de, Van De Voorde, S., Roeyers, H., Raymaekers, R., Oosterlaan, J., & Sergeant, J. A. (2009). How distinctive are ADHD and RD? Results of a double dissociation study. *Journal of Abnormal Child Psychology, 27,* 1007–1017.

Jonsdottir, S., Bouma, A., Sergeant, J. A., & Scherder, E. J. A. (2006). Relationship between neuropsychological measures of executive function and behavioral measures of ADHD symptoms and comorbid behavior. *Archives of Clinical Neuropsychology, 21,* 383–394.

Joyner, K. B., Silver, C. H., & Stavinoha, P. L. (2009). Relationship between parenting stress and ratings of executive functioning in children with ADHD. *Journal of Psychoeducational Assessment, 27,* 452–464.

Kaplan, B., Crawford, S., Cantell, M., Kooistra, L., & Dewey, D. (2006). Comorbidity, co-occurrence, continuum: What's in a name? *Child Care, Health, and Development, 32,* 723–731.

Kashani, J. H., McGee, R. O., Clarkson, S. E., Anderson, J. C., Walton, L. A., Williams, S., et al. (1983). Depression in a sample of 9-year-old children: Prevalence and associated characteristics. *Archives of General Psychiatry, 40,* 1217–1223.

Kashani, J. H., & Orvaschel, H. (1988). Anxiety disorders in mid-adolescence: A community sample. *American Journal of Psychiatry, 145,* 960–964.

Kendall, P. C. (1992). Anxiety and depression in children and adolescents. *Psychological Bulletin, 111,* 244–255.

Kertesz, A., Nadkarni, N., Davidson, W., & Thomas, A. W. (2000). The Frontal Lobe Inventory in the differential diagnosis of frontotemporal dementia. *Journal of the International Neuropsychological Society, 6,* 460–468.

Khalifa, N., & Knorring, A. von (2007). Prevalence of tic disorders and Tourette syndrome in a Swedish school population. *Developmental Medicine and Child Neurology, 45*(5), 315–319.

Korenblum, C. B., Chen, S. X., Manassis, K., & Schachar, R. J. (2007). Performance monitoring and response inhibition in anxiety disorders with and without comorbid ADHD. *Depression and Anxiety, 24,* 227–232.

Kurlan, R., Como, P. G., Miller, B., Palumbo, D., Deeley, C., Andersen, E. M., et al. (2002). The behavioral spectrum of tic disorders: A community-based study. *Neurology, 59*(3), 414–420.

Last, C. A., Perrin, S., Hersen, M., & Kazdin, A. E. (1996). Prospective study of childhood anxiety disorders. *Journal of the American Academy of Child and Adolescent Psychiatry, 35,* 1502–1510.

Leckman, J. F. (2004). Phenomenology of tics and natural history of tic disorders. *Brain and Development, 25*(Suppl. 1), S24–S28.

Lefkowitz, M. M., & Tesiny, E. P. (1985). Depression in children: Prevalence and correlates. *Journal of Consulting and Clinical Psychology, 53,* 647–656.

Lewinsohn, P. M., Hops, H., Roberts, R. E., Seeley, J. R., & Andrews, J. A. (1993). Adolescent psychopathology: I. Prevalence and incidence of depression and other DSM-III-R disorders in high school students. *Journal of Abnormal Psychology, 102,* 133–144.

Lewis, B. A., Freebairn, L. A., & Taylor, H. G. (2002). Correlates of spelling abilities in children with early speech sound disorders. *Reading and Writing: An Interdisciplinary Journal, 15,* 389–407.

Lezak, M. D. (1995). *Neuropsychological assessment (3rd ed.).* New York: Oxford University Press.

Lezak, M. D. (2004). *Neuropsychological assessment (4th ed.).* New York: Oxford University Press.

Loesch, D. Z., Bui, Q. M., Grigsby, J., Butler, E., Epstein, J., Huggins, R., et al. (2003). Effect of fragile X status categories and the fragile X mental retardation protein levels on executive functioning in males and females with fragile X. *Neuropsychology, 17,* 646–657.

Loh, P. R., Piek, J. P., & Barrett, N. C. (2011). Comorbid ADHD and DCD: Examining cognitive functions using the WICS-IV. *Research in Developmental Disabilities, 32,* 1260–1269.

Luman, M., Oosterlaan, J., & Sergeant, J. A. (2005). The impact of reinforcement contingencies on ADHD: A review and theoretical appraisal. *Clinical Psychology Review, 25,* 183–213.

Luria, A. R. (1966). *Higher cortical functions in man.* New York: Basic Books.

Mackie, S., Shaw, P., Lenroot, R., Greenstein, D. K., Nugent, T. F., III, Sharp, W. S., et al. (2007). Cerebellar development and clinical outcome in attention deficit hyperactivity disorder. *American Journal of Psychiatry, 76,* 647–655.

Mahone, E. M., Cirino, P. T., Cutting, L. E., Cerrone, P. M., Hagelthorn, K. M., Hiemenz, J. R., et al. (2002). Validity of the Behavior Rating Inventory of Executive Function in children with ADHD and/or Tourette syndrome. *Archives of Clinical Neuropsychology, 17,* 643–662.

Mahone, E. M., Hagelthorn, K. M., Cutting, L. E., Schuerholz, L. J., Pelletier, S. F., Rawlins, C., et al. (2002). Effects of IQ on executive function measures in children with ADHD. *Child Neuropsychology, 8,* 52–65.

Mahone, E. M., & Hoffman, J. (2007). Behavior ratings of executive function among preschoolers with ADHD. *Clinical Neuropsychologist, 21,* 569–586.

Mangeot, S., Armstrong, K., Colvin, A. N., Yeates, K. O., & Taylor, H. G. (2002). Long-term executive function deficits in children with traumatic brain injuries: Assessment using the Behavior Rating Inventory of Executive Function (BRIEF). *Child Neuropsychology, 8,* 271–284.

Mares, D., McLuckie, A., Schwartz, M., & Saini, M. (2007). Executive function impairments in children with attention-deficit hyperactivity disorder: Do they differ between home and school environments? *Canadian Journal of Psychiatry, 52,* 527–534.

Martel, M. M. (2009). Research review: A new perspective on attention-deficit/hyperactivity disorder: Emotion dysregulation and trait models. *Journal of Child Psychology and Psychiatry, 50,* 1042–1051.

Mash, E. J., & Barkley, R. A. (2003). *Child psychopathology* (2nd ed.). New York: Guilford Press.

Masters, J. C. (1991). Strategies and mechanisms for the personal and social control of emotion. In J. Garber & K. A. Dodge (Eds.), *The development of emotion regulation and dysregulation* (pp. 182–209). New York: Cambridge University Press.

Mattson, S. N., Goodman, A. M., Caine, C., Delis, D. C., & Riley, E. P. (2006). Executive functioning in children with heavy prenatal alcohol exposure. *Alcoholism: Clinical and Experimental Research, 23,* 1808–1815.

McAuley, T., Chen, S., Goos, L., Schachar, R., & Crosbie, J. (2010). Is the Behavior Rating Inventory of Executive Function more strongly associated with measures of impairment or executive function? *Journal of the International Neuropsychological Society, 16,* 495–505.

McGrath, L. M., Hutaff-Lee, C., Scott, A., Boada, R., Shriberg, L. D., & Pennington, B. F. (2008). Children with comorbid speech sound disorder and specific language impairment are at increased risk for attention-deficit/hyperactivity disorder. *Journal of Abnormal Child Psychology, 36,* 151–163.

Melnick, S. M., & Hinshaw, S. P. (2000). Emotion regulation and parenting in AD/HD and comparison boys: Linkages with social behaviors and peer preference. *Journal of Abnormal Child Psychology, 28,* 73–86.

Mervis, C. B., & John, A. E. (2010). Cognitive and behavioral characteristics of children with Williams syndrome: Implications for intervention approaches. *American Journal of Medical Genetics, Part C: Seminars in Medical Genetics, 154C,* 229–248.

Milich, R., Ballentine, A. C., & Lynam, D. R. (2001). ADHD/combined type and ADHD/

predominantly inattentive type are distinct and unrelated disorders. *Clinical Psychology: Science and Practice, 8*, 463–488.

Mitchell, J. T., Knouse, L. E., Nelson-Gray, R. O., & Kwapil, T. R. (2009). Self-reported ADHD symptoms among college students: Item position affects symptom endorsement rates. *Journal of Attention Disorders, 13*, 154–160.

Mitchell, M., & Miller, S. (2008). Executive functioning and observed versus self-reported measures of functional ability. *Clinical Neuropsychologist, 22*, 471–479.

Miyake, A., Friedman, N. P., Emerson, M. J., Witzki, A. H., Howerter, A., & Wager, T. D. (2000). The unity and diversity of executive functions and their contributions to complex "frontal lobe" tasks: A latent variable analysis. *Cognitive Psychology, 41*, 49–100.

Mulligan, A., Anney, R. J. L., O'Regan, M., Chen, W., Butler, L., Fitzgerald, M., et al. (2009). Autism symptoms in attention-deficit/hyperactivity disorder: A familial trait which correlates with conduct, oppositional defiant, language, and motor disorders. *Journal of Autism and Developmental Disorders, 39*, 197–209.

Murphy, K. R., & Barkley, R. A. (1996). Prevalence of DSM-IV ADHD symtoms in adult licensed drivers. *Journal of Attention Disorders, 1*, 147–161.

Newcorn, J. H., Halperin, J. M., & Miller, C. J. (2009). ADHD with oppositionality and aggression. In T. E. Brown (Ed.), *ADHD comorbidities: Handbook for ADHD complications in children and adults* (pp. 157–176). Washington, DC: American Psychiatric Publishing.

Nigg, J. T. (2006). *What Causes ADHD?* New York: Guilford Press.

Nigg, J. T., & Casey, B. J. (2005). An integrative theory of attention-deficit/hyperactivity disorder based on the cognitive and affective neurosciences. *Development and Psychopathology, 17*, 765–806.

Norman, D. A., & Shallice, T. (1986). Attention to action: Willed and automatic control of behavior. In R. J. Davidson, G. E. Schwartz, & D. Shapiro (Eds.), *Consciousness and self-regulation: Advances in research and theory* (Vol. 4., pp. 1–18). New York: Plenum Press.

Olfson, M., Marcus, S. C., Weissman, M. M., & Jensen, P. S. (2002). National trends in the use of psychotropic medications by children. *Journal of the American Academy of Child and Adolescent Psychiatry, 41*, 514–521.

Oosterlaan, J., Logan, G. D., & Sergeant, J. A. (1998). Response inhibition in AD/HD, CD, comorbid AD/HD+CD, anxious, and control children: A meta-analysis of studies of the Stop Task. *Journal of Child Psychology and Psychiatry, 39*, 411–425.

Oosterlaan, J., Scheres, A., & Sergeant, J. A. (2005). Which executive functioning deficits are associated with AD/HD, ODD/CD and comorbid AD/HD + ODD/CD? *Journal of Abnormal Child Psychology, 33*. 69–85.

Paloyelis, Y., Mehta, M. A., Kuntsi, J., & Asherson, P. (2007). Functional MRI in ADHD: A systematic literature review. *Expert Reviews in Neurotherapeutics, 7*, 1337–1356.

Pennington, B. F. (1997). Dimensions of executive functions in normal and abnormal development. In G. R. Lyon & N. A. Krasnegor (Eds.), *Development of the prefrontal cortex: Evolution, neurobiology, and behavior* (pp. 265–281). Baltimore: Brookes.

Pennington, B. F., & Ozonoff, S. (1996). Executive functions and developmental psychopathology. *Journal of Child Psychology and Psychiatry, 37*, 51–87.

Piek, J. P., Dyck, M. J., Francis, M., & Conwell, A. (2007). Working memory, processing speed, and set-shifting in children with developmental coordination disorder and attention-deficit hyperactivity disorder. *Developmental Medicine and Child Neurology, 49*, 678–683.

Pliszka, S. R. (2009). *Treating ADHD and comorbid disorders: Psychosocial and psychopharmacological interventions.* New York: Guilford Press.

Pontius, A. A. (1973). Dysfunction patterns analogous to frontal lobe system and caudate nucleus syndromes in some groups of minimal brain dysfunction. *Journal of the American Medical Women's Association, 26*, 285–292.

Popper, K. (1979). *Objective knowledge: An evolutionary approach* (rev. ed.). Oxford, UK: Clarendon Press.

Pribram, K. H. (1973). The primate frontal cortex: Executive of the brain. In K. H. Pribram & A. R. Luria (Eds.), *Psychophysiology of the frontal lobes* (pp. 293–314). New York: Academic Press.

Pulsifer, M. B. (1996). The neuropsychology of mental retardation. *Journal of the International Neuropsychological Society, 2,* 159–176.

Qian, Y., Shuai, L., Cao, Q., Chan, R. C. K., & Wang, Y. (2010). Do executive function deficits differentiate between children with attention deficit hyperactivity disorder (ADHD) and ADHD comorbid with oppositional defiant disorder? A cross-cultural study using performance-based tests and the Behavior Rating Inventory of Executive Function. *Clinical Neuropsychologist, 24,* 793–810.

Ranney, T. A. (1994). Models of driving behavior: A review of their evolution. *Accident Analysis and Prevention, 26,* 733–750.

Re, A. M., Pedron, M., & Cornoldi, C. (2007). Expressive writing difficulties in children described as exhibiting ADHD symptoms. *Journal of Learning Disabilities, 40,* 244–255.

Ready, R. E., Stierman, L., & Paulsen, J. S. (2001). Ecological validity of neuropsychological and personality measures of executive functions. *Clinical Neuropsychologist, 15,* 314–323.

Reddy, L. A., Hale, J. B., & Brodzinsky, L. K. (2011). Discriminant validity of the Behavior Rating Inventory of Executive Function parent form for children with attention-deficit/hyperactivity disorder. *School Psychology Quarterly, 26,* 45–55.

Reiersen, A. M., Constantino, J. N., Volk, H. E., & Todd, R. D. (2007). Autistic traits in a population-based ADHD twin sample. *Journal of Child Psychology and Psychiatry, 48,* 464–472.

Reynolds, C., & Kamphaus, R. (2004). *Behavior Assessment System for Children—2.* Circle Pines, MN: American Guidance Service.

Riccio, C. A., Hall, J., Morgan, A., Hynd, G. W., & Gonzalez, J. J. (1994). Executive function and the Wisconsin Card Sort Test: Relationship with behavioral ratings and cognitive ability. *Developmental Neuropsychology, 10,* 215–229.

Roberts, R. E., Attkisson, C. C., & Rosenblatt, A. (1998). Prevalence of psychopathology among children and adolescents. *American Journal of Psychiatry, 155,* 715–725.

Roessner, V., Becker, A., Banaschewski, T., & Rothenberger, A. (2007). Executive functions in children with chronic tic disorders and ADHD: New insights. *European Child and Adolescent Psychiatry, 16*(Suppl. 1), 36–44.

Rogers, S. J. (1998). Neuropsychology of autism in young children and its implications for early intervention. *Developmental Disabilities Research Review, 4,* 104–112.

Roth, R. M., Isquith, P. K., & Gioia, G. A. (2005). *Behavior Rating Inventory of Executive Function—Adult Version.* Lutz, FL: Psychological Assessment Resources.

Rowe, R., Maughan, B., & Goodman, R. (2004). Childhood psychiatric disorder and unintentional injury: Findings from a national cohort study. *Journal of Pediatric Psychology, 29,* 119–130.

Sagvolden, T., Johansen, E. B., Aase, H., & Russell, V. A. (2005). A dynamic developmental theory of attention-deficit/hyperactivity disorder (ADHD) predominantly hyperactive/impulsive and combined subtypes. *Behavioral and Brain Sciences, 25,* 397–468.

Schleepen, T. M. J., & Jonkman, L. M. (2010). The development of non-spatial working memory capacity during childhood and adolescence and the role of interference control: An N-back task study. *Developmental Neuropsychology, 35,* 37–56.

Schonfeld, A., Paley, B., Frankel, F., & O'Connor, M. (2006). Executive functioning predicts social skills following prenatal alcohol exposure. *Child Neuropsychology, 12,* 439–452.

Semrud-Clikeman, M., Walkowiak, J., Wilkinson, A., & Butcher, B. (2010). Executive functioning in children with Asperger syndrome, ADHD-combined type, ADHD-predominantly inattentive type, and controls. *Journal of Autism and Developmental Disorders, 40,* 1017–1027.

Shallice, T. (1994). Multiple levels of control processes. In C. Umilta & M. Moscovitch (Eds.), *Attention and performance XV: Conscious and nonconscious information processing* (pp. 395–420). Cambridge, MA: MIT Press.

Shallice, T., & Burgess, P. W. (1991). Deficits in strategy application following frontal lobe damage in man. *Brain, 114,* 727–741.

Shatz, D. B., & Rostain, A. (2006). ADHD with comorbid anxiety: A review of the current literature. *Journal of Attention Disorders, 10,* 141–149.

Shaywitz, S. E., Shaywitz, B. A., Fletcher, J. M., & Escobar, M. D. (1990). Prevalence of reading disability in boys and girls: Results of the Connecticut Longitudinal Study. *Journal of the American Medical Association, 264,* 998–1002.

Shelton, T. L., Barkley, R. A., Crosswait, C., Moorehouse, M., Fletcher, K., Barrett, S., et al. (1998). Psychiatric and psychological morbidity as a function of adaptive disability in preschool children with high levels of aggressive and hyperactive–impulsive–inattentive behavior. *Journal of Abnormal Child Psychology, 26,* 475–494.

Simonoff, E., Pickles, A., Charman, T., Chandler, S., Loucas, T., & Baird, G. (2008). Psychiatric disorders in children with autism spectrum disorders: Prevalence, comorbidity, and associated factors in a population-derived sample. *Journal of the American Academy of Child and Adolescent Psychiatry, 47,* 921–929.

Singer, H. S., & Walkup, J. T. (1991). Tourette syndrome and other tic disorders: Diagnosis, pathophysiology, and treatment. *Medicine (Baltimore), 70,* 15–32.

Sinzig, J., Walter, D., & Doepfner, M. (2009). Attention deficit/hyperactivity disorder in children and adolescents with autism spectrum disorder: Symptom or syndrome? *Journal of Attention Disorders, 13,* 117–126.

Skinner, B. F. (1953). *The science of human behavior.* New York: MacMillan.

Son, S. E., & Kirchner, J. T. (2000). Depression in children and adolescents. *American Family Physician, 62,* 2297–2308, 2311–2312.

Spencer, T., Biederman, J., Coffey, B., Geller, D., Wilens, T., & Faraone, S. (1999). The 4-year course of tic disorders in boys with attention-deficit/hyperactivity disorder. *Archives of General Psychiatry, 56,* 842–847.

Stavro, G. M., Ettenhofer, M. L., & Nigg, J. T. (2007). Executive functions and adaptive functioning in young adults with attention-deficit/hyperactivity disorder. *Journal of the International Neuropsychological Society, 13,* 324–334.

Stuss, D. T., & Benson, D. F. (1986). *The frontal lobes.* New York: Raven Press.

Swanson, H. L., & Jerman, O. (2006). Math disabilities: A selective meta-analysis of the literature. *Review of Educational Research, 76,* 249–274.

Tannock, R. (2009). ADHD with anxiety disorders. In T. E. Brown (Ed.), *ADHD comorbidities: Handbook for ADHD complications in children and adults* (pp. 131–155). Washington, DC: American Psychiatric Publishing.

Thomas, C. P., Conrad, P., Casler, R., & Goodman, E. (2006). Trends in the use of psychotropic medications among adolescents, 1994–2001. *Psychiatric Services, 57,* 63–69.

Thorell, L. B. (2007). Do delay aversion and executive function deficits make distinct contributions to the functional impact of ADHD symptoms? A study of early academic skill deficits. *Journal of Child Psychology and Psychiatry, 48,* 1061–1070.

Thorell, L. B., Eninger, L., Brocki, K. C., & Bohlin, G. (2010). Childhood Executive Function Inventory (CHEXI): A promising measure for identifying young children with ADHD? *Journal of Clinical and Experimental Neuropsychology, 32,* 38–43.

Thorell, L. B., & Nyberg, L. (2008). The Childhood Executive Functioning Inventory (CHEXI): A new rating instrument for parents and teachers. *Developmental Neuropsychology, 33,* 536–552.

Toren, P., Sadeh, M., Wolmer, L., Eldar, E., Koren, S., Weizman, R., et al. (2000). Neurocognitive correlates of anxiety disorders in children: A preliminary report. *Journal of Anxiety Disorders, 14,* 239–247.

Valera, E. M., Faraone, S. V., Murray, K. E., & Seidman, L. J. (2007). Meta-analysis of structural imaging findings in attention-deficit/hyperactivity disorder. *Biological Psychiatry, 61,* 1361–1369.

Vazsonyi, A. T., & Huang, L. (2010). Where self-control comes from: on the development of self-control and its relationship to deviance over time. *Developmental Psychology, 46,* 245–257.

Vloet, T. D., Konrad, K., Herpertz-Dahlmann, B., Polier, G. G., & Gunther, T. (2010). Impact of anxiety disorders on attentional functions in children with ADHD. *Journal of Affective Disorders, 124,* 283–290.

Vriezen, E. R., & Pigott, S. E. (2002). The relationship between parental report on the BRIEF and performance-based measures of executive function in children with moderate to severe traumatic brain injury. *Child Neuropsychology, 8,* 296–303.

Vygotsky, L. S. (1962). *Thought and language* (E. Hanfmann & G. Vakar, Eds. & Trans.). Cambridge, MA: MIT Press.

Walshaw, P. D., Alloy, L. B., & Sabb, F. W. (2010). Executive function in pediatric bipolar disorder and attention-deficit hyperactivity disorder: In search of distinct phenotypic profiles. *Neuropsychology Review, 20,* 103–120.

Warnke, A. (1999). Reading and spelling disorders: Clinical features and causes. *European Child and Adolescent Psychiatry, 8*(Suppl. 3), III2–III12.

Welsh, M. C., & Pennington, B. F. (1988). Assessing frontal lobe functioning in children: Views from developmental psychology. *Developmental Neuropsychology, 4,* 199–230.

Willcutt, E. G., Doyle, A. E., Nigg, J. T., Faraone, S. V., & Pennington, B. F. (2005). Validity of the executive function theory of attention-deficit/hyperactivity disorder: A meta-analytic review. *Biological Psychiatry, 57,* 1336–1346.

Wilson, B. A., Alderman, N., Burgess, P. W., Emslie, H., & Evans, J. J. (1996). *Behavioral Assessment of the Dysexecutive Syndrome.* Bury St. Edmunds, UK: Thames Valley Test Company.

Wolf, L. E., & Wasserstein, J. (2001). Adult ADHD: Concluding thoughts. In J. Wasserstein, L. E. Wolf, & F. F. Lefever (Eds.), Adult attention deficit hyperactivity disorder: Brain mechanisms and life outcomes. *Annals of the New York Academy of Sciences, 931,* (pp. 396–408).

Wood, R. L. I., & Liossi, C. (2006). The ecological validity of executive function tests in a severely brain injured sample. *Archives of Clinical Neuropsychology, 21,* 429–437.

Woodruff-Borden, J., Kistler, D. J., Henderson, D. R., Crawford, N. A., & Mervis, C. B. (2010). Longitudinal course of anxiety in children and adolescents with Williams syndrome. *American Journal of Medical Genetics: Part C. Seminars in Medical Genetics, 154C,* 277–290.

Youngstrom, E. A., Arnold, L. E., & Frazier, T. W. (2010). Bipolar disorder and ADHD comorbidity: Both artifact and outgrowth of shared mechanisms. *Clinical Psychology: Science and Practice, 17,* 350–359.

Zandt, F., Prior, M., & Kyrios, M. (2009). Similarities and difference between children and adolescents with autism spectrum disorder and those with obsessive compulsive disorder: Executive functioning and repetitive behavior. *Autism, 13,* 43–57.

Zito, J. M., Safer, D. J., dosReis, S., Gardner, J. F., Magder, L., Soeken, K., et al. (2003). Psychotropic practice patterns for youth: A 10-year perspective. *Archives of Pediatric and Adolescent Medicine, 157,* 17–25.

Index

Page numbers followed by *f* indicate figure, *t* indicate table